Listening

to

ADD

A Unique Perspective :
Management Strategies and Insight for People
with ADD and those who know them

By

Ian Provo MSW, LCSW

Foreword by Robert Eme, PhD

authorHOUSE™

1663 LIBERTY DRIVE, SUITE 200
BLOOMINGTON, INDIANA 47403
(800) 839-8640
WWW.AUTHORHOUSE.COM

First published by AuthorHouse 01/25/05

ISBN: 1-4184-9644-8 (sc)

Printed in the United States of America
Bloomington, Indiana

This book is printed on acid-free paper.

This book is for my parents and my wife, who have always stood by me.

And for Cameron.

FOREWORD

There is a remarkable international consensus that Attention Deficit Disorder (ADD) is a real disorder with characteristic symptoms that can be recognized and treated[1]. This may come as a revelation to some who recall disagreements about the nature of ADHD throughout the media. In fact: **All major medical associations and government health agencies assert that ADHD is a real developmental brain disorder**. These agencies include the U.S. Surgeon General, the American Medical Association (AMA), the American Psychiatric Association, the American Academy of Child and Adolescent Psychiatry (AACAP), the American Psychological Association, and the American Academy of Pediatrics (AAP). Furthermore, these experts not only recognize ADD as a valid disorder but also agree that we know a lot about it.

Real disorder means that there is overwhelming scientific evidence that something exists and that it causes serious impairments in major life activities such as education, occupational functioning, independent living, and social and family relationships. We know that ADD is a real disorder because existing scientific evidence has convinced virtually all the experts in the medical, psychiatric, and psychological professions that this indeed is so. Or, in the words of the commission organized by the American Medical Association in regard to various public concerns regarding ADD: *"ADD is one of the best researched disorders in medicine, and the overall data on its validity are far* *more compelling than for most mental disorders and many medical conditions,"*[2] with more than 1,000 scientific articles published on it every year. It also should be noted here that this real disorder, which is the most commonly diagnosed behavioral disorder of childhood (occurring in about 6 percent to 9 percent of a school-aged population), is not confined to childhood, but its significantly impairing symptoms persist into young adulthood for the majority of children with ADD.

Developmental brain disorder means impairment in certain brain functions that one is born with (genetics) that manifests itself as the individual develops.

Impairment means that certain brain functions, and hence, psychological mechanisms, are not functioning properly.

There may be a variety of types or subtypes of ADD or even different kinds of ADD. The type that this book deals with is characterized by symptoms that are predominantly inattentive without high levels of overactivity or impulsivity. Indeed, it is important to note that the predominantly inattentive type actually occurs more often than the type that includes overactivity and impulsivity.[3] This latter type, however, is more commonly diagnosed, especially among juvenile males because it causes more social havoc. Furthermore, as many as 85 percent of adults with ADD, and especially the predominantly inattentive type, have not been diagnosed[4] because the general public, as well as medical and mental health professionals, have not been properly educated on adult ADD. Hence, the value of Mr. Provo's book, which traces the development of an individual with ADHD into adulthood.

In addition, Mr. Provo provides many striking illustrations of classic symptoms of ADD that are frequently misunderstood. For example, one of the most harmful misunderstandings is that because the performance of those with ADD can be incredibly variable, the problem is simply one of *willpower.* For example, statements such as the following are legion when it comes to ADD.

My skin crawls when I have to sit down and study boring material. After 3-4 minutes I will tune out or fall asleep. It requires tremendous energy to stay focused. Consequently, I am a "deadly procrastinator." (Young adult male)

In my own personal experience, I suffered greatly throughout my education. I recall feeling frustrated since grade school. My boredom got the best of me; therefore, I began to dream. I believe boredom is tied to ADHD in that the person with ADHD learns to adapt to under stimulation by engaging in fantasy as a way of creating stimulation (Twenty-five-year-old female with a PsyD in psychology).

What these statements illustrate is that individuals with ADD have an impairment in sustained attention. This is the ability to stay on task and pay attention, especially to those activities which are repetitive, effortful, uninteresting, or are chosen for the individual by another. The classic example is that of homework. In most cases, dull, boring, mind-numbing homework is: never done, only partially done, done only when a person is constantly flogged by a parent to do so, or is done only at the last minute in a rushed, haphazard dash to the finish. However, in tasks they find interesting, persons with ADD can sustain attention for hours—a young person with ADD can play video games forever! Most individuals with ADD have a few activities where ADHD impairments are absent, which may make ADD look like a willpower problem, a problem of simple laziness. It is not![5]

The reader is encouraged to fully sustain attention to the following explanation. It addresses what is the single most damaging misunderstanding of ADHD. The incredible variability in the ability of individuals with ADD to sustain attention is not because they are any more lazy, irresponsible, or unmotivated than the person without ADD. It is because **THEIR BRAINS CANNOT SUSTAIN ATTENTION IN CIRCUMSTANCES THAT THEY FIND TEDIOUS, DULL, OR BORING**.

Studies of individuals with and without ADD illustrate brain patterns that highlight the differences in the brains of those with and without ADD. When faced with a tedious, dull, boring task, the brain regions engaged by the task of those without ADD are awake, aroused, activated; whereas, these same brain regions of those with ADD are under-aroused, under-activated.

Hence, for the time being, the message is simply this: Most people can make themselves sustain attention to boring tasks. Those with ADHD are gravely impaired in so doing because the brain regions that should enable them to do so are impaired. ADD is a disorder of brain impairment, not a disorder of laziness or willpower.

Try this analogy. You are very fatigued but you must continue to read this book, do your homework, and pay the bills. Certainly, you can vigorously and earnestly struggle against sleepiness and complete the task at hand. It will take a great deal more effort and more time than if you were rested and alert, but it is doable. Now imagine spending your entire life having to intensely struggle to sustain attention to the numerous tasks that you do not find invigorating. You would be at high risk for developing the unsavory reputation of a lazy, irresponsible, and unmotivated, etc. Welcome to the world of ADD!

Finally, another valuable contribution of Mr. Provo's book is that it wonderfully illustrates the fact that approximately 88 percent of those with ADD will develop another psychological disorder in their lifetime, largely as a result of having ADD. This is commonly referred to as *co-morbid* disorder, which simply means that another disorder co-exists with ADD. Mr. Provo's accounts of his anxiety and panic episodes are prime examples of co-morbidity.

In summary, Mr. Provo provides a wonderful developmental account of ADD that illustrates many aspects of a disorder that despite its common currency is still too often misunderstood.

Robert Eme, PhD.

[1]
R. Barkley, "International Consensus Statement Issued," *Clinical Child and Family Psychology Review* 5 (2002): 89-111.

[2]
L. Goldman and R. Bezman, "Diagnosis and Treatment of Attention Deficit/Hyperactivity Disorder," *Journal of the American Medical Association* 279 (1998): 1100-1107.

[3]
M. Reiff and S. Tippins, *ADHD: A Complete and Authoritative Guide* (American Academy of Pediatrics, 2004).

[4]
E. Hill, "Diagnosis, Evaluation, and Treatment of Adult ADHD" (Tenth Annual ADDA Conference, St. Louis, MO, May 13-16, 2004).

[5]
T. Brown, "Barriers to 'Demystification of AD/HD and Willpower'" (Tenth Annual ADDA Conference, St. Louis, MO, May 13-16, 2004).

Robert Eme, PhD, is Professor of Clinical Psychology at the Argosy University Illinois School of Professional Psychology, where he teaches coursework on Attention-Deficit Hyperactivity Disorder.

INTRODUCTION

Many books have been written on the subject of Attention Deficit Disorder (ADD). More recently, books have emerged describing the characteristics and features of this disorder in adults. However, unlike other books on this topic, this author offers a unique perspective from his firsthand experience of living with Attention Deficit Disorder.

Despite skepticism, ADD is a very real disorder. Many have argued that ADD is simply a disorder that has been created by professionals, doctors, and drug companies for the purpose of financial gain. Others would argue that the symptoms are "all in your head," or merely some manifestation of a self-fulfilling prophecy.

In a sense, it is fair to question a diagnosis of ADD, especially when there are so many other disorders whose symptoms mimic that of ADD. There are few qualified, trained professionals who can accurately diagnose ADD. Many professionals, although well meaning, do not understand the fundamentals of co-morbidity and are unable to distinguish the similar yet subtle differences between ADD and other disorders. Also, a diagnosis of ADD can often be a quick and easy explanation for a more complicated problem.

Another problem contributing to society's reluctance of accepting ADD as a legitimate disorder is that we are leery of blame and tired of excuses.

Many perceive those alleging a diagnosis of ADD as individuals who are lazy, malingering, avoid work, evade responsibility, or who are unwilling to take ownership of their actions. For those who genuinely suffer from this disorder, nothing could be farther from the truth.

As a professional, I have worked with both ADD children and adults. I have had the opportunity of lecturing in the community on this topic. However, despite my studies on this subject, review of the literature, and research of current data, I understand ADD for a very different reason. I *have* ADD.

Every day I face the challenges of living with ADD. I know what it's like to be repeatedly fired from employment and to experience debilitating feelings of low self-esteem. I empathize with those who have difficulty remaining focused and find concentration an arduous task. I understand what it is like to be distracted by the constant bombardment of environmental stimuli. I can appreciate the frustration of frequently misplacing items and the accompanying problems of short-term memory impairment. I have often walked into a room and forgotten why I was there.

As do many other individuals with ADD, I have learning disabilities. I know what it's like to fail academically. I have had teachers tell me that I am lazy. I inadvertently interrupt others. For me, procrastination is a hovering cloud and a haunting companion. I have difficulty with change. I quickly grow restless. I become bored easily.

Notwithstanding these symptoms, I have managed to survive and progress throughout life. I have had to develop my own life script, which is constantly being revised. I have, however, found common recurring themes, interventions, techniques, and solutions to approaching ADD. I have developed a set of coping strategies and insights that can aid individuals who are struggling with the daily battles of ADD. As I share my story of coping with ADD, I will tell you which interventions work and which interventions do not. I will explain to you the dos and don'ts of working with ADD children and adults.

The skills necessary to deal with ADD must be consistently practiced. A key to working with ADD children and adults is the development of insight. Insight itself is an acquired skill. There are neither quick fixes nor illusions in the treatment of ADD. Those peddling quick solutions or making fantastic claims of miracle cures are not being honest with themselves and are misrepresenting the very crux of the helping professions.

When considering ADD, we need to listen to what people with this disorder are saying. Conversely, people with ADD need to listen to what the disorder is saying; i.e., recognize its symptoms, and understand its meaning and its impact on routine life. If they listen well, those with the disorder may learn to manage it.

Through diligence, perseverance, and patience you *can* create an impetus for change. It is my hope that as the reader absorbs the information in this book, he or she will find inspiration, hope, and practical solutions for himself, a loved one, or someone else living with ADD.

TABLE OF CONTENTS

FOREWORD.. vii

INTRODUCTION xv

PART I Childhood...1
   CHAPTER ONE Into the World and On To
   School 3
   CHAPTER TWO A Gift Becomes a Curse.........11
   CHAPTER THREE A Recipe for Disaster 19

PART II Young Adult...39
   CHAPTER FOUR A Young Adult with ADD 41
   CHAPTER FIVE Another Disorder....................51
   CHAPTER SIX Continuing Education..............53

PART III Adulthood 63
   CHAPTER SEVEN The Denial Years.................65
   CHAPTER EIGHT Cruel Irony 77

PART IV Solutions 91
   CHAPTER NINE Devising a Game Plan...........93
   CHAPTER TEN Gaining Insight—The Big
   Risk 99
   CHAPTER ELEVEN Taking It Up a Notch.....107
   CHAPTER TWELVE Have a Sense of Humor 111
   CHAPTER THIRTEEN Interpreting and
   Accepting ADD..113

CONCLUSION **127**

EPILOGUE **135**

ACKNOWLEDGMENTS **137**

PART I

Childhood

CHAPTER ONE

Into the World and On To School

To fully appreciate my story, you must first understand the times in which I have lived. I was born in 1965 when the term "ADD" did not exist. From an early age, there were certain indicators suggesting that a problem existed. For the first eight to nine months of my life, I had frequent colic. I had hypersensitivity to certain tactile stimuli. I was a child who constantly tore the tag from his shirt collar. I was easily startled. I was restless and had fitful sleep. My mother describes a common, nightly occurrence in which, while down on all fours, I would rock back and forth in my crib. By morning, my crib would be on the opposite side of the room. The wooden floors made it easy for me to propel my crib across the room. Not knowing what to do, my parents had me assessed by a pediatrician. I was prescribed Phenobarbital, which in the 1960s was a common practice. The pediatrician also suggested that my parents keep very few items in my room, thus leaving as few stimuli as possible. That intervention was helpful. My chronic restlessness did, however, have a payoff. At age seven months, I was able to stand alone, and by eight months I walked everywhere.

The structure and dynamics of my family would have a profound impact on how teachers and professionals would interpret and react to my ADD. My parents are both highly educated. My father has a PhD from Stanford University and he taught foreign languages at a local college. He speaks several languages. My mother also holds advanced degrees in language and linguistics. I am the second child born into a family of four children. I have three sisters. I am closest in age to my oldest sister. We are eighteen months apart. In grade school she was primarily an A-student. In fact, all three of my sisters at one time or another had report cards with straight A's.

I learned to speak at an early age. I was able to read by the time I entered kindergarten. However, these gifts and talents would later become a curse. Teachers expected much from me but I could not meet those expectations. At the end of the first grading period, my teacher informed my parents that I had barely completed half of the required work. My parents were in disbelief. They knew that I could read. To them this didn't make any sense.

My teacher said, "Ian would do fine if he would just stop daydreaming." She also said, "Ian just doesn't pay attention in class." My parents would ask me, "If you're not doing your work during class, then what *are* you doing?" My response was always the same: "I don't know?" I didn't know. I didn't have the slightest clue as to how much time I spent in class "spacing-out." However, the biggest challenge I would face was learning to write. I simply could not keep up with the rest of the class. It took every ounce of concentration

I had just to put together a four-word sentence. I remember the intense frustration I felt as I attempted to put words on paper. My writing was illegible and my spelling incomprehensible, and in a dyslexic manner I often inverted my letters.

Worst of all this was the homework. During the 1970s in my school district, the academic standard of measure was based on one's ability to complete purple ditto sheets, a product of the antiquated mimeograph machine. Some of you may remember these purple ditto handouts. If nothing else, you may remember the cheap high one could get from sniffing their fumes. If having ADD didn't cause you to "space-out," the fumes from the purple ditto sheets certainly would. Because I wasn't completing the work in school, all the work that I didn't complete was sent home. Again, because I couldn't stay with any task for more than five or ten minutes, the concentration required for writing down answers was overwhelming. In the evening as I sat at the kitchen table, I would pound the table with my fists and clench my teeth, in a vain effort to finish my work. The academic focus was always on the quantity of completed ditto sheets, while the quality of the work was far less significant.

Upon entering the second grade, I discovered that my teacher had a great intolerance for "slow learners." On my first-quarter report card, she made the following comment: "Ian is capable of doing better, but he is so slow getting things done." I soon learned that she had a greater intolerance for disorganization. One day, while lifting up my desktop, my teacher gazed into my desk and observed an abyss of disarrayed papers, very characteristic of an ADD child's desk. She responded by giving me a hard slap on my back. On another occasion, while I was "daydreaming," I felt a sudden, loud, hard slap to the back of my head. Apparently this form of discipline was meant to cure me of my symptoms. I doubt that it cured me of anything, but I did learn that teachers were to be feared and not to be trusted.

Third grade offered new challenges. My mathematical learning disability was now in full bloom. My third-grade teacher, however, did not believe in physical discipline as a means of correcting my poor performance. Her method of choice was abject humiliation. When I did poorly on a math assignment, instead of explaining my mistakes and offering suggestions for improvement, in front of the entire class, she tore my paper to shreds and threw it in the wastebasket, declaring, "This is no good!" My parents were livid.

In 1972 there were no 504 laws or Individual Educational Plans for disabled students. There were no grievance procedures or legal recourse for parents if a school failed to provide adequate accommodations for a student. Children with learning disabilities had no rights. My mother certainly was unaware of any student rights. She attended grammar school in Great Britain during the 1940s. To her, the mistreatment and humiliation of children was commonplace. My father sought help from a colleague who was employed as a professor of psychology at the same college where he taught. I was tested. It was concluded that, *"There was indication of slight constitutional basis for tiring or satiating more readily than typical for age."* No one, including the psychologist himself, was actually sure what that meant, but this was the first time that there was actual documentation substantiating that I had an impairment. The school, however, was not impressed.

My parents provided the school with a number of suggestions that might help me improve my performance. They first suggested that I be given more time to complete examinations. They then requested that I be allowed to take some of the tests by oral examination. They knew, as did I, that my written work was not an accurate representation of what I really knew or understood. Oral testing would be one means by which I could demonstrate my knowledge of the subject matter. Finally, my parents suggested that it would be in everyone's best interest if the standard of measure applied to grade my performance focused more on quality than on quantity. I then might be able to succeed. These suggestions were quickly dismissed and ultimately rejected. Apparently, the school enjoyed its voluminous output of purple ditto sheets, and besides, as it was explained, "It wouldn't be fair to the other children."

The fourth grade offered new hope. I was assessed by my pediatrician and was given a formal diagnosis of "Minimal Brain Dysfunction." I was started on a trial regiment of Ritalin. The Ritalin was helpful. More importantly, I had a teacher who was willing to work with my parents and my pediatrician. He maintained regular contact with both. Rather than holding firmly to rigid, traditional forms of assessment, Mr. Nelson was flexible and willing to explore different approaches to my education.

My parents never pressured me to perform, nor did they place a strong emphasis on getting high grades. They knew my strengths and my weaknesses. My pediatrician made a profound observation regarding my self-esteem. He said, "It doesn't matter if you don't pressure Ian about grades. He knows that he's in a family of achievers." He was right. I knew that I was inherently different from my parents and my sisters. For parents, it is important to note that ADD children *know* that they are different. They are keenly aware that they do not measure up to their peers. To further complicate this problem, ADD children have no idea as to why they're not the same. I remember being genuinely perplexed and puzzled as to why I could not perform as well as the other students, and I was very aware that my three sisters were getting straight A's and I wasn't. Why couldn't I get straight A's, or any A's at all?

Even if parents encourage and compliment their ADD child to enhance his self-esteem, e.g., "You can do it! You're smart and I believe in you," the child often does not believe what he is being told. Too often parents fall into a false sense of security, believing that their repeated compliments will eventually eliminate any self-esteem issues. In my professional work, I have often heard parents exclaim, "But we always tell him how smart he is." "That's a good start," I explain, "but your child won't believe you until he experiences it for himself." Do not, however, let this deter you from making complimentary statements of assurance, confidence, and capability. It was ultimately these types of statements that pulled me through some of my darkest moments. I continued to succeed because I was repeatedly told that I *would* succeed. If you're going to create a self-fulfilling prophecy for a child, make it one of success.

CHAPTER TWO

A Gift Becomes a Curse

One of the disadvantages of having educated parents, specifically a father who was a college professor, is that everyone else expected me to perform at a gifted and accelerated level. My oldest sister had also paved the way for high expectations, with her straight A's and quiet disposition. I was a very articulate child, and for my age had an advanced vocabulary, one of the benefits of having two linguists in the home. I could hold intelligent conversations with adults. My teachers, however, would use this gift against me. To them, my gifted speech and ability to articulate only served as proof of how truly lazy I must be. "Anyone that smart just isn't trying." That reasoning would hound me for the rest of my academic career. I would often hear statements like, "I'm surprised you don't know that Ian. Your father is a college professor!" My sixth-grade teacher once said to my mother, "I wish Ian could be more like Michele" (my oldest sister). She broke the number-one rule of parenting and teaching: *Never compare one child to another.*

I experienced a significant event in the fifth grade. Up to that point, no teacher had actually failed me or given a grade lower than a C. For whatever reason, between the first through fourth grades, I was spared from that experience. I had certainly performed at a level where I could have easily been given an F. That would all change. As I opened my second-quarter report card, I saw a series of lettered grades. Almost all of them were D's. I was shocked and in disbelief! I was overcome with emotion and began to cry. Steve, my best friend, asked me what was wrong. I was too embarrassed to give specific details other than that I had done poorly on my report card.

That negative experience was an important event. For the first time, I realized that I would be held accountable for any work I did not complete. It was a rude awakening—innocence lost. In order for me to fully comprehend natural and logical consequences, I needed the experience of receiving failing grades. No longer could I slide by through the grace and mercy of my teachers. If I gave up and shut down, my grades would plummet.

In fifth grade, my grades would fluctuate from one extreme to another. During one grading period, I received an A in reading. That was then followed by two grading periods of straight D's. This vacillation of grades is common among ADD children and adults. Many ADD children and adults energetically approach a project with every intention of completing it within the required time frame. However, one of the heavy burdens of ADD is that this level of enthusiasm diminishes quickly. I was no exception. My road to completing homework was paved with good intentions. I would start off each quarter similar to a recovering addict. "This time I'm really going to work the program" or "I can get good grades any time I want." Of course that wasn't true. As soon as I began to feel any level of comfort, I would let down my guard and return to a chronic pattern of procrastination. Learning to recognize and identify that pattern is difficult for any child.

Of all the ADD symptoms I have, the biggest proverbial "thorn in my side" is that of impairment in short-term memory. In school, this impairment was obvious. I was the kid who was known for always leaving his sack lunch at home. On a fairly regular basis, my mother would appear outside my classroom door holding my lunch. It became such a regular event that other students could quickly recognize my mother approaching from several blocks away. I would often hear, "Hey Ian, I see your mom, and she's bringing your lunch." Another living nightmare was that of losing pencils (now replaced by pens). I don't know of anyone who went through as many packages of pencils as I did. I often wonder how many forests had to be cut down in order to replace the pencils that I had lost. I'm surprised that Green Peace never picketed or protested outside my home.

At home, I would misplace articles of clothing, toys, homework, money, and other items. I would also forget to bring home my homework assignments. More often than not, I would simply deny that I even *had* any homework. Do not assume that your ADD child intentionally wants to lie about not completing his homework. A better explanation is that the child is overwhelmed, and so far behind in his work that he or she may feel too embarrassed or ashamed to admit his dilemma. Harsh criticism and parental retribution may be feared. A raised voice and harsh criticism are the worst possible responses a parent can give an ADD child. Whenever I received a D or failed a subject, my parents never had to say anything. I felt bad enough. I was already struggling with low self-esteem and depressed feelings. Any negative feedback from my teachers regarding my grades served no practical purpose. Lecturing as a means of *correcting* ADD behaviors does not work. Never add insult to injury.

In my profession I have seen many parents employ punitive measures in an effort to "get him to realize the importance of getting his work done." "Believe me," I would reply, "after all the punishment he's received, I'm sure he understands perfectly well the importance of completing his homework." The problem here is that the parent (or teacher) falsely assumes that punishing an ADD child will condition him to complete all of his homework, similar to shocking a rat trapped in a maze. This logic and reasoning does not work because the problem with ADD is that the deficiency lies within the very same brain that you are trying to condition. If the ADD child also has a learning disability, you then have two areas of the brain that are not functioning correctly. Behavior modification may be used effectively to correct acting-out behaviors, but it is a poor tool when used as a means to improve comprehension and academic performance. In many schools, clear distinctions are made between students who have a learning disability

(LD) compared with students who are behaviorally disordered (BD). On occasion, the two may overlap, but ADD should be viewed first as a learning impairment. Therefore, the educational plan for an LD child should be different from the educational plan for a BD child.

Another common mistake regarding ADD and behavior modification is the parents' reliance on cause-and-effect thinking. When a child behaves impulsively, he's not thinking about consequences. All bets are off. ADD children take longer to comprehend and then assimilate the concepts of natural and logical consequences. For these reasons, when compared to their peers, ADD children often require a higher degree of supervision.

For the purposes of this book, I have used the term "ADD" synonymously with "Inattentive Type," "Predominantly Hyperactive Type," and "Combined Type." I have the predominantly Inattentive Type of ADD. Children who are more outwardly hyperactive are usually the first to catch their teacher's attention, i.e., "the squeaky wheel gets the oil." It is the inattentive type of ADD children who are most likely to fall through the cracks. They are often overlooked by educators and dismissed as being "slow" or "lazy." The Hyperactive types of ADD children are often quickly labeled as a "troublemakers" Other children who *are* problematic but do not have ADD are often targeted as "needing to be on Ritalin." For these reasons, mental health professionals often refer to ADD as the most over-diagnosed yet under-diagnosed disorder.

As I completed grammar school, not much had changed in respect to my grades and my ability to function in the classroom. When taking Ritalin, I had a feeling of being "zoned-in" as opposed to being "zoned-out," a sensation that is difficult to describe. I remember feeling an almost intense rush of concentration. Ritalin did not help my learning disability, but it did play a positive role in helping to improve my concentration in school. Unfortunately, the side effects from the medication became unbearable. When taking Ritalin, I suffered from frequent and intense headaches. As a child I was always thin and underweight. Ritalin completely obliterated my already poor appetite. With Ritalin, proper weight maintenance was seriously threatened. My pediatrician eventually discontinued its use.

Regardless of my personal experiences of taking Ritalin, I am a strong advocate of using medication to treat ADD. First of all, it would be important to note that the extreme side effects from my Ritalin usage were the exception and not the norm. Secondly, there are now numerous other medications in addition to Ritalin that effectively treat ADD symptoms. Many of the newer drugs have even fewer side effects.

In fairness to Ritalin, before condemning its usage, acquaint yourself with the facts about this drug. Opponents of Ritalin question its safety and long-term usage. To date, Ritalin has been studied more than any other psychostimulant in history. Its efficacy and safety has been well established. Although Ritalin is classified as a psychostimulant, it is not addictive. Ritalin stimulates the area of the brain that is not being sufficiently stimulated. Ritalin is slow acting, without creating a "high," unlike cocaine, which causes an immediate release of Dopamine into the brain. Studies have shown that children who take Ritalin are less likely to abuse drugs as adults. Less than 1 percent of individuals who are prescribed Ritalin will ever demonstrate addictive symptoms. Always talk with your physician regarding any concerns you may have about taking stimulant medication. Get the facts.

CHAPTER THREE

A Recipe for Disaster

I was not even remotely prepared for middle school. Middle school has to be one of the *worst* possible settings for an ADD child. Instead of having only one or two teachers, the student now has seven or eight. The student also has seven or eight different classes located in seven or eight different rooms, with seven or eight different textbooks. The ADD student is assigned a hall locker and gym locker, and has to remember the combinations to both. I couldn't even remember where I last placed my pencil; how was I going to remember different rooms, numerous textbooks, and locker combinations?

I had another problem that faces all children at one time or another: *peer acceptance*. Being the shortest male in the school did not help matters, and consequently I was an easy target. I was mercilessly teased and bullied. Observing that I was of small stature, some kids thought it amusing to, at a high rate of speed, run up to me and then slam me up against my locker or flat onto the ground. While running laps around the gym, sometimes someone would intentionally trip me. Children can be cruel.

I heard a lot of the same criticisms and complaints from my middle school teachers that I had heard from my grade school teachers. Many scoffed at the idea that I had a learning disability. Some of the teachers had had my sister Michele in their class. Others knew of my father and his status as a college professor. I was continually told that I was lazy and that I should have superior performance in the classroom because, "Your father is a college professor."

I began experiencing anxiety. I became overwhelmed with homework, antagonistic peers, and critical teachers. I was failing four courses. In those days, teachers handed out failure notices that were printed on bright pink paper. And, as was the custom, these failure notices were given to you in front of all the other students. The bright pinkness of the paper left no question as to which students were failing the class. It was then our responsibility to take the failure notice home to our parents, have them sign it, and then return it the following day. I rarely gave my parents failure notices, but kept them hidden. Shame and embarrassment prevailed over logic. My parents weren't going to punish me; they never had. That didn't matter. As previously stated, for some children, not meeting perceived expectations is the worst punishment of all. I was equally as critical of myself as others were. In my world, I was stupid and had failed my parents. One day I came home from school with four failure notices. The anxiety was too much for my mind and body. Later that evening, I experienced a series of frightening physical symptoms accompanied by an intense fear that I was going to die. Although, I didn't know it at the time, I was having a panic attack. I never told my parents about the panic symptoms or the failure notices. Not discussing the panic symptoms would be a mistake that would come back to haunt me.

Without providing me a single accommodation, the school now had a new message for me: "You're never going to make it in high school." This message was repeated to me many times. Parent-teacher conferences were no less comforting. My parents were told that perhaps they should prepare for the inevitability that I may not even *finish* high school. I had not even finished the seventh grade and I was already being written off as a lost cause. One teacher believed in me: Mr. Kohl. He wrote in my yearbook, "To Ian, a person loaded with potential." I had done poorly in his class, but he knew of my struggles and sensed my natural abilities. He spoke with my parents on a number of occasions. He liked me and I liked him. Sometimes, a teacher's positive comments can leave an indelible mark.

In middle school, I began to test my teacher's limits and boundaries. I had a math teacher who used a very unique catchphrase. If a student didn't complete an assignment due to not understanding the material, her response would always be, "I feel sorry for you, and my heart bleeds for you." This phrase was repeated numerous times. I finally responded by declaring, "Sounds like you have a serious heart condition. Maybe you should see a doctor." The other kids in the class laughed, but I found myself having to share that observation with the assistant principal. ADD children are at greater risk for seeking attention through nonacademic methods. I acted out because I felt acceptance from peers, and my behavior was one of the few things left in school that I could control.

My best friend Steve attended the eighth grade with me. The previous year he had attended an alternative middle school program. Having Steve near by was a blessing. Although I was short in stature, he wasn't. He helped deter a few bullies. Most of the previous year's bullies had moved on to high school. I tried to befriend the few remaining bullies, with limited success. I enjoyed the friendship of several girls, some of whom I had crushes on. There were some days when I actually looked forward to going to school. I took a communications class that involved mostly oral presentations. I got an A. That was a huge boost to my self-esteem. Math, however, would continue to be a problem.

Through diligence and perseverance, my parents were able to get me into a resource math course. There were only three other students in the class. I received a lot of one-on-one attention. The math was being taught at about the fourth- or fifth-grade level. At the end of the quarter, I received a B. The school concluded that since I had done so well in the remedial class, I no longer needed to be there. I was moved back into eighth-grade algebra. I flunked. Some foolish people had reached a foolish conclusion.

For some people, math is not that difficult. Certain individuals have an innate knack for solving equations.

To these people math makes perfect sense. From my perspective, math makes no sense at all. When discussing words and concepts such as irony, anarchy, supply and demand, urban warfare, and photosynthesis, an individual is able to give very concrete and specific examples of those definition and ideas. They can be easily defined and illustrated. Solving algebraic equations, however, requires using an entirely different part of the brain. I never completely understood the whole concept of adding letters, e.g., $a + b = y$. I'm not exactly sure for what reasons a person would want to solve for y. I knew that *pi* was *3.14* only because I had memorized it. To this day I have no idea what *pi* is or what function it serves. My purpose here is not to criticize math and the mathematical sciences, but to help the reader understand that when an individual has a mathematical learning disability, the brain functions of linear thinking and computational problem solving are impaired. While you are quickly drawing a conclusion to the problem's solution, the disabled individual is drawing a blank. I was always impressed with how quickly my friend Steve could whip out the answers to his math homework. He knew of my mathematical impairments, but like all good friends he just accepted the fact that "you suck at math."

In theory, I was now ready to begin high school, certainly an unexpected event, since I had already been told that I would never make it to high school. Somehow I did. I faced the inevitable dilemma of once again being the shortest person in school. Only this time I was in a school with approximately 1,600 other students. There were some advantages and disadvantages to being short. On the one hand, I received a lot of attention from juniors and seniors who were genuinely intrigued by my height. They would tease me, but this was always done in a fun-loving manner. They weren't being cruel, and, when passing through the halls, they would always say hello. If I was lucky, I would get an occasional hello from a cheerleader. On the other hand, there were still bullies in school, and the first day of school offered no immunity. I took a drama class. During the first day of class, I noticed that there were two other boys in the class who were making fun of me. One of them began to taunt me. I decided that I was not going to be intimidated and stood my ground. After the boy threatened me with bodily harm, I sarcastically retorted by stating, "Like I'm so scared." I *was* scared but I didn't want him to know that. Later that day, as I leaned against a wall eating my lunch, I was blindsided by a kick to the head. As I stared up from the ground, I saw the boy from my drama class. "You don't have such a smart mouth now, do you?" he exclaimed. Some of those same seniors and juniors who had befriended me had witnessed the entire event. Smallest kid in the school versus a real big kid; didn't seem fair to them. Suffice it to say, that boy would never bother me again.

Persons with ADD *can* and *will* often speak without thinking. The impulsivity that accompanies this disorder can have deleterious consequences. My mouth would get and has gotten me in trouble more times than can be counted. The sudden instance of frustration coupled with not knowing how to employ the "think-before-you-speak" rule is an ADD hardship. People can be offended by inappropriate comments made at inappropriate times. Interrupting others and speaking out of turn also presents challenges. When an ADD person has strong, passionate ideas, thoughts, or feelings, he may feel motivated to articulate those thoughts without first checking his social and environmental surroundings. Missing social cues, the individual may speak while someone else is speaking. He may also speak out of context, or, in other words, what he is saying has nothing whatsoever to do with topic of conversation. I learned about this *faux pas* through trial and error, and I also learned from the repeated feedback of peers, teachers, professionals, family, and friends. Eventually I started to pay attention, making sure that I would hold my tongue no matter how excited or angry I was feeling. I had developed insight. I still face this challenge on a daily basis. I am far from perfect but I still keep practicing. To develop that skill, one *must* practice.

My vacillation of grades continued throughout high school. I would go from one extreme to the other. For example, in freshmen English my grades for the four grading periods were, F, B, F, and B. I continued getting D's and was lucky if I could maintain a C average. I was excused from taking ninth-grade math because teachers concluded that "Ian just isn't ready." In those days, only one credit hour of math was necessary to fulfill the requirements for high school graduation. I would wait until my sophomore year before enrolling in General Math. As a sophomore, I continued taking drama and other classes that focused less on mathematics. I faced teachers who, like previous instructors, were convinced of my laziness. And the new catchphrase was, "You're never going to get into college!" One teacher in particular believed that my fluctuation in grades was a manifestation of passive-aggressive behavior.

I have worked with parents of ADD children who truly believed that their child was trying to spite them. "When he wants to do the work, he can do it!" or, "He's been told a hundred times to pick up his clothes; he remembers to do it only when he wants to remember!" they would argue. There is some truth to this argument but very little accuracy. For most people, motivation is not a light switch that can be tuned on and off at will. This especially holds true for children and adults with ADD. The argument that an ADD child or adult can "do the work if wants he wants to" has no merit. It is a false assumption to believe that the ADD child actually has internal control over motivation. There is also the dilemma of the child's having every intention of *wanting* to complete the task but not having the ability to follow through with what has been requested. Short-term-memory impairment then becomes the icing on the cake.

I never cease to be amazed at the number of people who claim that an individual who is capable of watching hours of television cannot possibly have ADD. Watching television is a *passive* activity. The television does all the thinking for you. Studies have shown that the brain waves of a person watching television are uniquely different from those of an individual who is engaged in some other activity. In fact, most people, whether they have ADD or not, find watching television soothing. Some ADD children and adults use television as a means of relaxation. If used appropriately and in moderation, television can be a useful tool for ADD children and adults.

In school, I was motivated by interest and ability. To create interest, teachers and parents should constantly be exposing children to a variety of subject matters. Their minds should be consistently challenged and awakened. If you can create a spark of interest, that in turn becomes a catalyst for motivation. When I became a junior in high school, I took a debate class and joined the debate team. That was a very good decision and had positive repercussions. I excelled in debate. On more than one occasion, I took home a first-place tournament trophy. I won two speech awards coming in first and second place. This did wonders for my self-esteem. Another positive outcome from being on the debate team was that I developed fundamental research skills. I would use those skills later in life. Ironically, one of my lowest GPAs was during the same grading period in which I took debate. People with ADD will often put all their time and effort into the one activity that interests them while neglecting other important tasks and assignments. Although I got an A in debate, during that same grading period I also received D's in English, science, and history. ADD children and adults must be taught how to balance activities, manage time, and prioritize tasks. I will discuss this further in a later chapter.

Winning debate awards helped me to wrestle with the internal demons of self-doubt. I began to believe that I actually stood a chance of being accepted into a college or university. I still had one big hurdle to leap: I had to pass a math class. I enrolled in General Math. Despite the difficulty, I persisted and put forth my best effort. One of the chapters in our textbook dealt with memorizing a few simple geometry formulas. We were tested on the memorization of the formulas and their application rather than actually being required to solve an equation. I was always good at memorization and consequently got my first and only A on a math exam. I still had one battle remaining: the final exam. As the teacher passed out the final examination, I sat at my desk and humbly offered my standard, ritualistic prayer: "Yea, though I walk through the valley of the shadow of math I will fear no evil. Thine is the equation and story problem forever, Amen." Deliverance, however, would come with a price. Because I had done well on one or two exams and had always turned in my homework, my teacher would pass me, while overlooking the biggest blunder of all: I had flunked the final exam.

There was one consolation that resulted from flunking my math final. My parents were insistent that I be given a series of diagnostic and aptitude tests. The school acquiesced, agreeing to test me. They also agreed to do a case study. The results were astounding.

There was a large discrepancy between my verbal and performance scores. This was especially true with math. Plotted on a graph, the drop in my performance ability looked something like the 1929 stock market crash. There it was in black and white. It couldn't be ignored. At seventeen years of age, as a junior in high school, I was officially recognized as "Learning Disabled" and, as provided by law, was entitled to all rights, services, and privileges. The school and its team developed my Individual Educational Plan (IEP). The plan said very little, if anything, other than agreeing that I had a disability. In regards to the ADD, my parents were told not to worry and that I would, "grow out of it." In response to the notion that an individual outgrows ADD, my parents have said, "That's the biggest lie we were ever told." In the early 1980s, people still believed that ADD was more or less a temporary condition. That belief would prevail well into the 1990s, and I am amazed at how many mental health professionals are presently teaching this archaic concept.

My senior year brought about a desire to develop better study habits. Keep in mind that I still had episodes where I would receive a B only to be followed by an F the next quarter. I enjoyed some semblance of a social status. I had a locker right next to the senior class president and enjoyed some of the perks associated with his locker being in such close proximity to mine. By this time, many of the students knew of my prowess in debate and drama. I had many friends, and like many high school students, I enjoyed a variety of activities.

My best friend Steve would largely influence the career path that I would choose. Steve, like me, had sisters but no brothers. He excelled in math, electronics, and computers. I, on the other hand, excelled in language and arts. In that respect, we complemented each other. Although I could never seem to secure a girlfriend, Steve *always* had one. The problem with Steve, however, was that his relationships were always unhealthy. Somehow, Steve managed to hook up with girls who were "really messed up" (to use a less clinical term). Whenever he got into an argument with one of his girlfriends, I would take on the role of the peacekeeper. His girlfriends would come to me for sympathy and feedback. I would listen to them and offer simple advice. Eventually, I began noticing patterns. Some of these girls came from dysfunctional families where abuse and alcoholism were common. Consequently, many had serious issues with self-esteem, voiced suicidal ideation, and in retrospect were most likely clinically depressed.

Steve would always get sucked into these unhealthy dynamics. Although I didn't know it at the time, I was inadvertently developing rudimentary counseling and assessment skills. Thank you, Steve.

Two teachers would also contribute to solidifying my vocational path. Mr. Sbragia taught sociology. No one surpassed his teaching method. He was vibrant, energetic, and erudite. He told colorful stories to illustrate sociological concepts and ideas. More importantly, Mr. Sbragia had tremendous faith in the human potential. He always complimented his students.

He devoted entire lesson plans to the teaching and understanding of self-esteem. He taught the importance of healthy communication and emphasized that people should always be told that they are of value and worth. He practiced what he taught. He showed me a more visually based note-taking method, a technique that I would continue to use throughout my life.

Mrs. Guarino taught psychology. She brought the subject to life. After taking her class, I was convinced that I wanted to pursue a career in the mental health profession. Her class was one of the few classes in which I received an A. A "successful" report card was one that contained no D's, and such report cards were rare.

I was still worried that without algebra, I might not be accepted into college. At my own insistence, I made two unsuccessful attempts at passing an algebra course. In order to apply to any college, I would have to take the ACT. I took the exam and scored especially well in the social sciences. The math section of the ACT was a complete fiasco. In math, my cumulative score was three. My performance in English was marginal. I was disheartened with my final ACT score, especially knowing that it was my math rating that had negatively impacted my overall score, one of the few mathematical concepts that I actually understood. Nevertheless, the day had finally arrived when I walked across the stage and received my high school diploma. I had survived high school and would now have to face the world as an ADD young adult, and I was ill prepared to do that.

Ian Provo MSW, LCSW

HELPFUL SUGGESTIONS AND INSIGHTS
for parents, teachers, and professionals

1. *Never compel an ADD child to finish his homework right after school.* Children, like adults, need downtime. ADD children need time to relax and unwind. Some children come home from school exhausted and overwhelmed. Give them space.

2. *When doing homework, offer short but frequent breaks.* Staying on task is difficult for any ADD child. Let the child get up, get a drink, use the bathroom, and *then* have him return to the task.

3. *Ask for a reduction in the amount of homework being assigned.* Something is inherently wrong when a parent must spend the entirety of each and every evening engaged in assisting his child in completing homework. If such is the case, you have every right to approach the school and request a modification in your child's curriculum. In some instances, homework can be altogether eliminated. No parent or child should have to live a life where every waking hour is a continuation of school.

4. *Plan for change.* Remember, even the slightest disruption in schedule or routine can unnerve the ADD child. This would include, but is not be limited to, changing seating assignments, lunch schedules, moving furniture to another area of a room, having a new teacher, etc. If you know that such a change is to occur, discuss it with

the child beforehand. Walk him through the process and reassure him of his well-being.

5. *Plan for forgetfulness.* Many ADD children will consistently forget to bring certain items to school. The child's memory must become reliant on visual cues. For example, if a child forgets to bring his lunch to school, the lunch should be placed directly in front of the door. The idea here is that the child cannot leave the house without picking up his lunch. Brightly colored Post-It notes can also augment visual cues. For example, if a child forgets to wear his glasses to school, a reminder note can be posted on the bathroom mirror, followed by the glasses then being taped to the door. A second note can also be posted on the door. I have had parents report great success using this kind of intervention. I can attest that this works equally well with adults. Schools can also implement the use of visual cues.

6. *Make learning a multisensory experience.* ADD children effectively learn through multiple stimuli. Always use visual aids. Make learning a tactile, hands-on experience. Provide a variety of activities that will foster and enhance personal growth and learning.

7. *Identify your child's strengths.* Every child has certain gifts and talents. Your responsibility as a parent is to help your child identify what those gifts are. Expose your child to music, art, literature, sports, and cultural events. Let him join clubs, groups, or organizations that

mentor children and that will encourage them to explore and pursue hobbies and interests.

8. *Make your child's self-esteem the first priority.* In order to feel good about themselves, all children must experience some measure of success. To create such an experience, the parent and school must first provide the child with realistic goals. Whenever a child succeeds in a task, behavior, or assignment, the parent (or school) should immediately identify the progress and praise the child accordingly. Remember to give the child specific and concrete examples of how he has succeeded. Always point out to the child that what he has achieved signifies improvement and demonstrates capability. Praise and praise again.

9. *Know the laws and know your rights.* Familiarize yourself with student educational rights. Every school district must provide information on how to request services for children who could potentially qualify for special eligibility. Consult with educational advocates and surrogates. Know and understand "due process." Check websites for local school policies and support groups.

10. *Be a team player.* Remember, when working with the schools, an adversarial approach does not work. Be diplomatic. Anger and other reactive behaviors only create defensiveness. You are an integral part of your child's educational team. Attend all staffings. Be flexible and make compromises. If necessary,

maintain daily contact with the school. If new issues arise, then request a staffing. Put all your requests in writing and submit a copy to both the teacher and the principal. Make copies of everything.

11. *Teach your child about ADD.* In the simplest terms, parents should educate their child about his disorder. If explained in clear and specific language, children are able to grasp the fundamentals of ADD. For example, a parent might say, "You're very smart, but sometimes your mind and body move too quickly. It is also hard for you to remember things. Sometimes you have difficulty paying attention in class because you're thinking about lots of other things. This medicine will help your mind and body to pay attention better." Give the child more information coinciding with his cognitive development.

12. *Do not give your child more than one or two directions at a time.* ADD children and adults do not do well with multiple tasks. If your child is getting ready to go to bed, do not ask him to brush his teeth, get dressed, and lay out clothing for the next day. Ask him to first brush his teeth. Only when he has finished that task should you ask him to do something else. Remember, one task at a time.

13. *Always be specific.* This is especially true when asking a child to correct behaviors. Don't say, "Be good at school," but instead say, "Don't talk to your neighbor when the teacher is

talking," or, "Please keep your hands and feet to yourself." Vague requests are open for interpretation. Avoid that mistake.

PART II

Young Adult

CHAPTER FOUR

A Young Adult with ADD

After high school, I would be accepted into a junior college. The college was located in the southeastern corner of Idaho. It was a private college run by the same church of which I am a member. However, before I could go to college, I would need a summer job. My self-esteem would hamper my efforts at securing employment. Although I had graduated from high school, I lacked confidence. I was afraid of failure and genuinely believed that I was not capable of holding or maintaining employment. Most of the jobs in our area would require the use of a cash register, something that scared me to death.

I was an immature eighteen-year-old. I was naïve and, like many eighteen-year-olds, I thought I knew everything—a bad combination. I was also unaware of the significant financial responsibility required to attend college and survive in the adult world. I lacked sound judgment. As a result of this mindset, I would end up doing only a few odd jobs the entire summer. The rest of my education would have to be financed through the infamous government student loan program.

As summer came to an end, I packed my belongings and ventured out West to the great state of Idaho. Moving away from home, I would face my first big phase-of-life adjustment. People with ADD have difficulty with change and I epitomized that symptom. Nobody hated change as much as I did. I liked everything just the way it was. Throughout my life, I had resisted any degree or measure of change. If I came home from school and someone had rearranged the furniture, repositioned the television, changed the curtains, or was sitting in "my chair," I would come unglued. I relied heavily upon consistency and routine. It became such a problem that my parents and sisters would, in advance, all forewarn me of any impending change. They would have special family meetings "just for Ian." During that meeting, I would be presented with the forthcoming change, e.g., "We're getting new drapes." We would then process my feelings about the new drapes. My oldest sister would then humorously but forcefully state, "We're getting new drapes, so get over it." After the new drapes arrived, I would then be debriefed. This process would be repeated as needed. My family was quick to instruct my wife on the effective use of this technique. Occasionally, we still have to have one of those "special meetings."

I was now living in a small Idaho town, 1,400 miles from home. It was a difficult adjustment. On the first day of classes, while engaging in foolish horseplay, I suffered a severe sprain to my left knee. I would spend the first month of college using crutches and wearing a knee brace. I made friends but was wrought with homesickness. I attended all my classes but my heart was not into studying. The magnitude of change was overwhelming. It would take me about three months to settle into my new environment. I lived in a noisy dormitory and had a roommate who was intrusive and controlling. He was critical of my lifestyle, music, friends, study habits, etc. At night, this roommate kept the windows open, making sure that the room always stayed cold. I frequently argued with him. As the only boy in the family, my bedroom had always been my sanctuary. I no longer had that luxury but now lived in what seemed like an Antarctic biosphere, with TV's *Frasier* for a roommate.

With incredible accuracy, the high school achievement test taken during my junior year predicted that during the first semester of college, I would most likely maintain a 2.0 GPA. My report card consisted of straight C's. Not impressive, but all passing grades.

I came home for Christmas and returned two weeks later to complete the spring semester. I did not want to return. I felt tremendous anxiety at the thought of having to once again be away from my family and friends. I had enjoyed spending part of the two-week break with my friend Steve. I could always count on him for comic relief, as he shared the same prowess for mischievous behavior as I did. I was disappointed with my grades and vowed a better performance the following semester.

When I returned from winter break, I was given a new roommate. Much to my relief, Doug was very laid-back and had a pleasant disposition. This reduced the stress within my living environment. During the spring semester, I was registered for courses that were part of my social work major curriculum. These classes were more interesting than some of the general-education requirements that plague most college freshmen for the first several semesters of their academic careers. I did well in my social work and psychology classes. In order to satisfy the requirements for completion of a degree, I would need to pass a science class. Falsely assuming that I could breeze through the course, I registered for an introductory course in physical science. Unfortunately, in our textbook, there were many chapters that dealt with chemistry and physics equations. I would receive a D in that class.

I had less homesickness, but at times I felt its incapacitating effects. It is very typical for most college freshmen to go through an adjustment period as they begin a new life away from home. With ADD, that adjustment period can drag on for many months. The problem is that the ADD student never really comes to terms with the reality of the changes. Rather than having a sense of finality and accepting his situation, the student maintains a continuous state of resistance. That's exactly what I did. I focused most of my time on returning home rather than embracing the academic opportunities. By the semester's end, I was desperate to leave Idaho. The winter had been unusually cold, and snow fell as early as the last two days of summer and continued to fall well into spring. In October, I had experienced an earthquake, and by December I was lucky to have walked away from a car accident that, for all practical purposes, could have ended my life.

After experiencing my own private Idaho, I returned to Illinois. This time I would need a *real* summer job. Steve would save me from an exhaustive job search. Prior to returning home, I had telephoned Steve, who indicated that he was now the assistant manager of a local fried chicken establishment. I had a job waiting for me. Again, the thought of employment was frightening. It took me a little longer to learn all the aspects of my job, but I did make my debut as a fried chicken cook. I mixed batters, breaded chicken, and cooked fried mushrooms, livers, gizzards, and fries. My best friend was now my boss, which required a period of adjustment. However, when Steve wasn't working, the store manager was. My self-esteem would be tried to its limits. This man could yell. He was like a drill sergeant. If you weren't completely demoralized by the end of your shift then he hadn't done his job. The store manager demanded perfection. Any flaw or perceived flaw on my part would be met with a furious tongue-lashing. Memories of angry, critical teachers quickly resurfaced. Those negative reminders brought about self-doubt. I would come home from work feeling horrible, convinced that any day, I would be terminated.

I wasn't terminated, and eventually we saw very little of the manager, as he now spent all of his time opening a new store.

I have always been involved in my religion, attending church on a weekly basis and participating in the church youth group. From a very young age, I had decided that at age nineteen, I would serve a mission for my church. Throughout my life, my religion has always been a constant support. That summer, I was working in preparation for my mission, and after its completion I would return to school. Friends and family were supportive of this decision. I submitted all the appropriate paperwork and waited for a response. I would be assigned to serve an eighteen-month mission in the Philippines. I was very excited. I learned everything that I could about the Philippines. I studied all the materials that as a missionary I would need to know. I then left the United States and, from the San Francisco airport, flew to the Philippines.

As the plane reached its final approach, peering out the window I noticed a heavy mist covering the thick jungle foliage. Walking off the plane, the tropical heat hit me like a furnace blast. The jungle's pungent odor permeated the air. Things were no longer familiar. The Tagalog language was now the dominant tongue. I did not speak Tagalog but I would learn enough of the language to survive. In fact, I welcomed the challenge of learning a foreign tongue. I had been raised to embrace cultural diversity. I was now the minority in a country whose citizens had a beautiful, brown skin tone, complemented by rich, black hair. Like me, Filipinos are also short in stature. I would often here comments like, "Hey, 'Joe,' you're Filipino size," and after being in the country for several weeks, I was beginning to believe that my name really *was* Joe.

One day it began to rain. For the next nine days, without a break, the rain would fall. The continuous rainfall was depressing. I began to feel the sharp pangs of culture shock, and once again I was horribly homesick. I didn't speak the language and could not tolerate the food. The homesickness became crippling. I could not fathom the concept that I would not be home for Christmas and that I could not simply pick up the phone and call my friends and family. I was going to be in the Philippines for eighteen months, period. When I was at college, there was always a light at the end of the tunnel, as I knew that summer break was just around the corner. To relieve stress, I had any given number of recreational outlets available. As a missionary, I had rules and I couldn't do as I pleased. A two-week vacation was not an option.

These variables did not mix well with my ADD, especially since I was a person who barely tolerated change. Every familiar point of reference and avenue of security had now been removed. I was also being bombarded with a plethora of sights, smells, sounds, and sensations, all of which were unfamiliar. Everything was different. Nothing was the same and I wasn't coping. As the heat of day attacked me, perspiration would coat my skin. My stomach was sick and fragile. Already thin, I was losing weight. At night, I began to have the same frightening physical symptoms that I had experienced in the seventh grade: I was beginning to have panic attacks. The mission proved too much. Having been in the Philippines less than four months, I returned to the United States. When I returned home, I barley tipped the scales at ninety pounds. My emaciated appearance shocked my parents. The idiosyncrasies of my ADD were a key factor contributing to my inability to serve in the Philippines. My church was not at fault and certainly the loving people of the Philippines were not to blame. Persons with ADD must learn to place blame accordingly and accept the fact that sometimes nobody's at fault. Blame itself solves nothing.

Upon returning home, I felt humiliated, defeated, and guilty. On Sunday, when I attended church, what would people say when they saw me? I became wrapped in feelings of failure. I believed myself to be a big disappointment. I knew that I would return to school but I did not want to go back to Idaho. I was determined to apply to another western university. But like many people with ADD, my thinking was absolute and inflexible. I wasn't looking at the big picture. I had made up my mind that I would only attend a specific western university and there could be no other. I did not consider other options and had no backup plan. This kind of tunnel vision is an enemy to ADD sufferers. Many persons with ADD often fail because they stubbornly hold to one belief system. Consequently, I did *not* get accepted into the university of my choosing. Who was I kidding? Did I honestly believe that I would be admitted with my ACT scores and most recent GPA? I had applied to a university that required higher numbers than I could provide. I learned from the experience, but now felt more worthless than ever. What was I going to do? Where would I go to school? These questions would haunt me.

After a period of grieving, I went back to the drawing board. I searched through several college catalogs, looking for colleges located in warm but dry climates. I hated the cold and more recently had a dislike for humidity. I looked specifically at each of the university's social work programs. I spoke with an acquaintance of my mother who had an MSW from Arizona State University. He spoke highly of the undergraduate social work program. I was sold. I applied to the university and was subsequently accepted into the program. That would be the best academic decision of my life.

That summer, I worked at the same college where my father taught. I worked in the food services center, serving on the cafeteria food-line, catering weddings, banquets, and class reunions, and washing dishes. I worked all summer and saved my earnings. Financially, I was ready to leave. Emotionally, I felt tentative and unconfident. My thoughts were often poignant, and wrought with the usual feelings of self-doubt and failure.

That August I flew to Arizona. The desert topography was beautiful. The sun shone every day. The university was friendly and inviting. The campus atmosphere was relaxed and casual. It was 1985, Reagan was president, thin ties were in, and the group A-ha had a number-one hit song, "Take On Me." I was a sophomore at Arizona State University in Tempe, Arizona, and this time I was determined not to be defeated. I was angry. I had nothing to lose and everything to prove. The memory of past failures would drive and motivate me. I decided that no matter how I felt or what I experienced, I *would* graduate from this university. I quickly discovered the university's disabled student services. I provided appropriate documentation, and my entitlement to disabled services was recognized. This university had the most ADD-friendly environment that I had ever encountered. I could pick and choose from a wide variety of courses. For the first time, I didn't have to take all my classes at the crack of dawn. I made sure all my classes met in the late morning or early afternoon.

Generally speaking, college is far more ADD-friendly than high school. It's more like an independent study program. You're allowed to work at your own pace, and nobody will reprimand you if choose not to attend class. For someone with my type of ADD, ASU was the perfect environment. I had good roommates, one with whom I continue to maintain contact. I made many friends within my academic program. I attended study groups and had a regular study partner. More importantly, my grades reflected my newly found motivation. For the first time ever, my report cards consisted of mostly A's (but not straight A's). I was dumbfounded. How was it that I had gone from being a C-student to an A-student? Maturity was definitely a factor, although in many ways I still considered myself an immature young adult. Once I got my first A, I was addicted. The possibility of getting straight A's had actually become a reality. Over time, I would develop excellent study skills and reading habits. Iron will had driven me to succeed.

CHAPTER FIVE

Another Disorder

I would return home every summer and continue working for the college food services center. I enjoyed being home with family and friends. I would, however, face a new challenge. The panic attacks that I had experienced in the seventh grade, and then again in the Philippines, would return. As I had done before, I told no one about the attacks. I was too afraid. How was I going to describe what was happening to me if I didn't even understand what was happening? Describing symptoms of a panic attack to someone who has never had such an attack can be difficult. Imagine the most frightened you have ever been and then magnify that feeling twenty times. Now imagine feeling faint, nauseated, having numbness and tingling in your arms and other extremities. You begin to shake. The anxiety you feel is beyond anything that you have ever experienced. Your racing heart and accompanying chest tightness make it very difficult to breathe. Eventually you vomit. These were the types of symptoms I was having. Over time, I would begin to make associations concerning the locations and places where these attacks would occur. If I had an attack at a restaurant, the next time that I returned to that restaurant, I would fear having another attack. That fear would be enough to trigger an attack. Eventually I would avoid all restaurants. The panic attacks occurred in many locations. Over time I developed a condition known as *agoraphobia*. There were few places remaining where I could go without having a panic attack. I was incapacitated.

I stubbornly refused to tell my friends what was happening to me. I spoke with the same person who had introduced me to the ASU social work program. He explained that I probably had panic disorder and that I definitely had agoraphobia. I was resistive to the concept of taking medication. I had had this condition for nearly two summers, before I eventually saw a doctor and agreed to take medication. Within two weeks of taking the medication, I had been given back my life. I could go anywhere I wanted without having an attack. I enjoyed 100 percent freedom of mobility. Ironically, these attacks did not interfere with my education. Returning home exacerbated the symptoms of the disorder. At school, the symptoms were negligible.

CHAPTER SIX

Continuing Education

During the last semester of my junior year, the unthinkable happened. I had reached an educational hallmark. Of my own volition, I had gotten an A in every course; straight A's. I was ecstatic. How did that happen? I now had more faith in my educational abilities. It was another big boost to my self-esteem. That experience would prepare me for my final year at ASU. However, I would be quickly humbled by the reality of my learning disability. In order to fulfill the requirements for my degree, I would have to pass a statistical research course. My mathematical skills were that of a fourth-grader's. How was I going to pass a statistical research course? Arizona State University's disabled student services would come to my aid. They provided the university with updated aptitude scores and other data regarding my math deficiencies. They petitioned the social work board, requesting that I be allowed to take a qualitative research course in lieu of a statistical research course. After reviewing the petition, the board accepted my request and allowed me to make the substitution.

I went on to complete my senior year at ASU, and the boy whom teachers had said might not even complete high school graduated with his Bachelor's Degree in Social Work. I felt as though a huge burden had been lifted from me. It was a happy time in my life. I now began the difficult task of finding a professional job. I would work for one more summer in food services. At the beginning of the fall, I was offered a job at the local community mental health center. I worked for a brief period in Crisis Intervention until I could be transferred to Rehabilitation Services, the position for which I was originally hired. When I was a student, I had worked a two-semester internship with a mental health agency in Phoenix, so working with patients suffering from mental illness was not foreign to me. What was foreign was the idea that I was now responsible for the management and oversight of client files and the completion of all accompanying paperwork. When I worked in Crisis Intervention, there were indicators that my ADD was alive and well. It took me twice as long as the next staff member to fill out forms and complete documents. I often forgot the order and sequence of specific procedures. I misplaced paperwork and would forget to write appointments or deadlines on my calendar.

The Rehabilitation Services Department did not require much paperwork, but to my peers, it was obvious that I lacked self-confidence and had no idea as to how to take initiative in my work. One of my co-workers took an immediate disliking to me. For the first month or so, she said nothing. Then one day during lunch, she let fly with a barrage of criticisms. She made multiple observations regarding my ineptness on the job. She then said, "And you don't even have any friends" (I did). It was a scathing attack. I didn't know what to think but I knew that I was not happy working in an environment with that level of animosity. I'm sure that some of her issues were relevant, specifically concerning my ineptness. I know that my ADD symptoms played a role in how others perceived my professional competency. And let's face it, I was just out of college and still had a lot to learn. That experience would be a foreshadowing of future events. I had a colleague who once told me that "when you have ADD, it can bring out the worst responses from people." My defensiveness would become a personal obstacle. Persons with ADD can often be defensive, but there is a reason for this reaction. When you spend most of your life feeling criticized, real or perceived, you eventually develop a defense mechanism that will protect you from ownership and responsibility. Taking ownership and responsibility means having to once again admit to failure. I had an excuse and explanation for everything. That was how I learned to survive. The defensive ADD individual often does not realize that others perceive him that way. People with ADD must be taught how to recognize defensiveness.

I decided that I would go back to school and work towards the completion of my master's degree. As much as I had enjoyed attending ASU, I wanted to be closer to home and out-of-state tuition had become too costly. I would pursue my graduate studies at the University Of Illinois in Urbana/Champaign. Once again, I thrived in the college environment. The social work program was outstanding and I was able to put all my effort into studying, as I had saved enough money from my previous job so that I would not have to work while attending school. I made many new friends. My professors were very personable and the completion of a statistics course would not be required of me. The School of Social Work offered coursework that would allow me to continue specializing in mental health. Something negative did result from my academic successes. I had created a façade. Over time I began to deny the seriousness of my ADD.

Eventually, I deluded myself into thinking that I truly had outgrown ADD.

Before completing my master's degree, I would face one final, academic and personal challenge. I would have to complete a full-time internship. Because I was unable to secure an internship within my own city, I would have to move to another part of the state. As was typical, I was emotionally and financially ill prepared for such a move. I moved to the town where I would complete my internship. I moved there at least one month earlier than was necessary. As a result of this impulsive decision, I quickly ran out of money. The facility for which I worked had not even approved my contract. I would wait nearly two months before receiving my first paycheck. When I did receive it, it was too late. My car had broken down and I had no money in my bank account. There was tension in the home of the family from whom I had rented a room. With no money, I was unable to go home for weekends or drive down to Champaign. Panic attacks resurfaced, but this time without the agoraphobia. I began to feel excruciating pain in my left arm and shoulder. My arm tingled, and red blisters formed on my skin. A physician diagnosed me with shingles. I would get to go home after all. There were no medications for shingles, so my recovery would be long and painful. An ADD decision resulted in an ADD consequence. I was learning things the hard way. I always did.

I completed the internship and graduated from the University of Illinois with a Master's Degree in Social Work. I now had I to make more choices and decisions. Had I learned from my life's experiences? Would I do things differently if given a second chance? Yes and no. Like many adults and children with ADD, instant gratification supersedes logic and reasoning. Sometimes it takes numerous failures before the individual gains insight. For me, that was always the case.

HELPFUL SUGGESTIONS AND INSIGHTS
for ADD Adults

1. *Avoid absolute, black-and-white thinking.* Stay away from cognitive distortions that use words like *I can only, I must, I'll never, I have to,* and *it's absolutely necessary.* Remember, don't create unnecessary internal pressure. There is more than one way to achieve a goal. Don't stubbornly hold to only one way of looking at a problem. Regarding personal goals, time is relative. Do not subject yourself to unrealistic time frames. If something doesn't go as planned, it's not the end of the world. The sun will still rise on the following day.

2. *Change is.* Change is an unavoidable, inevitable reality. Prepare for change. If you know that you are going to encounter any kind of personal or environmental change, then learn everything you can about the impending change. For example, before moving to a new job, school, or apartment, visit the new location. Talk to individuals about the new location. Meet the individuals with whom you will be working, living, or otherwise associating. If an unexpected change occurs, don't freak out. Embrace the change and repeatedly remind yourself that change is good. The French have a saying: *Plus c'a change, plus c'est la même chose* (The more that things change, the more they stay the same). Intentionally change your routine. Force yourself to do things differently.

3. *Like yourself.* Don't become your biggest enemy and critic. Be fair to yourself. Recognize that even small accomplishments are a sign of progress. Do not compare yourself to others. There will always be people who excel in areas where you may be weak. Don't let that discourage you. Let it inspire you. Sometimes weaknesses can later become strengths. Don't internalize criticism.

4. *Consider counseling.* If you struggle with self-esteem or related depressed feelings, then find someone with whom you can share your feelings. A trained professional can assist in helping you process your feelings, offer guidance, and help you to develop and implement healthy coping strategies. This would also include finding a support group. Check the Internet for local CHADD organizations.

5. *Avoid blame and assume ownership.* This is especially difficult when you may feel that you are always being criticized for mistakes. Learn to separate fact from feelings. If something is your fault, be willing to admit responsibility. This does not mean that you have to beat yourself up over every mistake you make. Everybody makes mistakes. Admitting a mistake is a strong indicator of maturity. Looking for blame and finding fault in others will not diminish your ADD symptoms. If something is not your fault, then you need not take ownership. Ownership and blame are very different. Learn to recognize the difference.

6. *College students should ask for help.* If you qualify for services due to ADD or some other kind of learning disability, then you should utilize the services that are being offered. Some colleges and universities may require you to be retested or will ask you to provide current documentation regarding your disability. If you think that you may have ADD but are not sure, then have your physician refer you for an assessment. Student counseling centers can also be an assessment resource.

7. *Think before you act.* Be proactive and not reactive. Never let the intensity of emotions and feelings dictate your actions. Stop and think. Do not make capricious and arbitrary decisions. If a decision is made impulsively, without consideration for consequences, it will most likely be met with many difficulties. Before taking action, ask for another opinion and feedback from others. For example, you would not buy a house without first looking inside, nor would you buy a car without taking it for a test-drive. Never confront someone in anger. Wait until you have had time to think.

8. *Create a secondary memory.* One of the hallmarks of ADD is frequent forgetfulness. When you can't rely on your own memory, then you must develop a means by which you can recall important tasks, events, and assignments. There is no wrong way of doing this. Whatever works for you *is* the right way. A Palm Pilot or PDA (personal digital assistant) is an amazing

tool. It's like having your memory in your pocket. Some people always keep a notebook on their person so that every task can be written to paper. Post-It notes are great visual cues. The use of large, visual calendars is an effective memory tool. Portable Dictaphones can instantly store your words onto tape for immediate recall. If you have a friend who is willing to prompt and remind you of tasks, then that also can be an effective memory-recollection aid.

9. *Know your symptoms.* Although certain symptoms are common to ADD, it is important to become familiar with your most problematic symptoms. For example, while one individual with ADD may be able to screen out background noise, for another person with ADD, background noise may be a constant distraction. Prepare yourself for such situations. If you know that you can't work in a noisy environment, then close doors, turn off the television, and unplug the phone.

10. *Consider medication.* Adults with ADD can take medication. Some people falsely believe that psychostimulant medication is only for children because "it doesn't work with adults." Not true. In fact, I have heard many adults report great success when taking medication for their ADD symptoms. For some, many of the symptoms are completely eliminated. Speak with your physician if you think that you might benefit from medication therapy.

Ian Provo MSW, LCSW

PART III

Adulthood

CHAPTER SEVEN

The Denial Years

The future was now filled with limitless possibilities. With a Master's Degree in Social Work, I was ready to conquer the world. Would the world be ready for me? At that time, all three of my sisters were living out West. Two of them were now married. My friend Steve was also married. I was at an age when dating and eventual marriage were of utmost importance. My sisters suggested that if I had any chance of finding a significant other, I would fare much better out West. They knew of my poor track record in Illinois. I accepted their proposal and once again moved out West. And while staying true to character, I once again, on short notice, moved without having sufficiently planned for the event. I had not saved up enough money, had no job, and had nowhere to live. I would first stay with my oldest sister and then live with my youngest sister (much to their husbands' delight).

Before I could be hired, I would have to become licensed as a social worker in the state where I was now living. I had somehow overlooked that small detail. I would have to pass a licensure exam, and then submit a thick application packet to the state. It would take several months before I could even begin to look for work in my field. This is yet another example of how I had still not learned from my impulsive mistakes. I had moved, but no matter where I lived, the ADD was coming with me.

I got my social work license but would be turned down for several jobs, as other applicants were more qualified than I was—a humbling experience. I was eventually offered a position as a child abuse investigator—a huge mistake. I was elated to have found employment but I had no idea regarding what I was about to face. To fully appreciate this error, a closer examination of the word "investigator" is warranted.

An investigator is someone who must have a knack for paying close attention to detail. I had ADD; paying attention to detail wasn't exactly my strong point. But I wasn't thinking about ADD anymore. As far as I was concerned, that troublesome part of my past was ancient history. This job would require thorough follow-up skills. The state had established rigid timelines in which an investigation must be completed. The ability to meticulously document would also be an essential job function. It wouldn't be long before the Department of Investigations figured out that I was not the right man for the job. A co-worker had warned me of the impending termination. After my six-month probationary period, I was let go for "substandard performance." I appealed the decision, not because I had ADD or a learning disability but because when I was first hired, the director complained that I was "too short and looked too young" to be an investigator. I couldn't accept the fact that my job performance was the real issue. My appeal went nowhere. Apparently *size* is not a protected class, something that I should have learned from middle school. *Strike one.*

No big deal, I'll just find another job. Because I had been a state employee, I was able to find another job through the Department of Mental Health. I was offered a position at the state mental hospital. When I was in graduate school, I had spent a summer working at a local psychiatric hospital. This population was very familiar to me. The hospital was scenically located on the side of a mountain, offering a beautiful panoramic view of the valley below. One of the benefits of this job was a small caseload. The position offered a more hands-on approach in the treatment of the patients. My direct involvement with the patients kept me focused. The paperwork was minimal. I was part of a clinical team and presented cases every morning. My clinical skills began to sharpen and supervisors commended my verbal case presentations.

Occasionally, I would long to return to Illinois. Within a year, all three of my sisters had moved out of the area. I felt abandoned. Valentine's Day brought more misery. A girl, whom I liked and had consensually kissed, returned all of the roses and Valentine gifts that I had given her. On Sunday morning, when I went to retrieve the newspaper, there in front of my door were all my gifts. A note was attached: *"Dear Ian, this is all a big mistake."* While she was thinking about the F-word, "friend," the ADD part of my brain had already moved on to the M-word, "marriage." However, within two months of the Valentine's Day Massacre, I met the woman who would later become my wife. I had spent my entire life hearing the same response whenever I would try to take a friendship to a serious level: "It'll ruin the friendship," I was told. "Well, then let's ruin the friendship," I would argue. This time my friend would be my wife.

My wife had married someone with ADD. She had no idea what was to become of her life. She knew that I had an education and a good job. I was able to offer a plausible explanation as to why I had been "let go" from my position as a child abuse investigator. Like many people with ADD, I quickly became restless. Because I had achieved my goal of finding a wife, there was no further reason for me to continue living out West. Without much convincing, my wife agreed that it might be nice to move back to Illinois and away from the state where we currently resided. We packed our belongings and moved. Of course I had no job waiting for me. We did have some money, and my wife was able to rapidly secure employment.

It would take me several months to find a job. I was offered a position at the same agency where I had worked with my bachelor's degree. This time I was hired as a child and family therapist. I worked with many children who, like me, had ADD. Maintaining healthy boundaries with my clients, rarely in my career did I disclose my own childhood struggles with the disorder. I certainly was able to empathize with these clients.

Within six months of being hired, problems with my ADD began to emerge. My caseload began to grow. The larger the caseload, the more unmanageable it became. Once again, I was in over my head. I made excuses for the lateness in completing my work. For my six-month evaluation, my supervisor gave me a rating of *"poor."* He was very methodical in his work. He never missed a thing. As time passed, I became more defensive. I had more excuses and began to challenge and resist his authority. During this time, I had reached another professional milestone. I had completed two years of post-graduate work and passed my clinical board exam. I was now a licensed clinical social worker (LCSW). In the state of Illinois, that credential held many rights and privileges. On our team, there was only one other colleague who shared that status. In my mind, the LCSW was the end-all and be-all of my career. I foolishly believed that with this credential, I was now invincible. After all, LCSWs were highly sought after. Surely I was immune from termination. Who in his right mind would fire an LCSW? My supervisor was not impressed and quickly referred to this credential as "a piece of paper." Tension continued to build as I fell further behind in my paperwork. Eventually I would be given a "corrective action plan" for my poor work performance. This write-up would be one of many that I would receive in my career.

At some point, the management concluded that it was time for me to go. Every facet of my work became scrutinized. Sadly, I learned that even in my profession, dishonesty existed. To ensure a timely termination, management would go so far as to backdate the alleged sequence of my performance issues. By giving me three separate write-ups on the same day but assigning a different date to each one, management could create the illusion of a progressive disciplinary process where none existed. A meeting was held in the personnel office, where I was the guest of honor. I was scolded and then fired. LCSWs *could* be fired. My departure was humiliating. In front of other staff, security stood over me as I packed my belongings, and then they escorted me out the door. *Strike two.*

To further add insult to injury, this agency tried to block my attempts at filing for unemployment. They argued that I had engaged in "willful misconduct" because on more than one occasion they had warned me about my considerable backlog of paperwork. An employment hearing was held. My wife and father were in attendance. The hearing officer concluded that nothing I had done fit the definition of "willful misconduct." I would get an unemployment check. During the hearing, I was grilled by my former employer. My father declared, "My son has ADD." I was horrified and embarrassed. "That has nothing to do with anything," I emphatically responded. I was still in denial. My father knew that ADD was the primary reason for my inability to complete the required paperwork.

ADD is not "willful misconduct." Mental health supervisors falsely believed that my poor work performance was a deliberate and willful attempt to spite their authority. More importantly, a new and erroneous misconception was beginning to unfurl. *People employed within the mental health profession should not have ADD.* The words of my colleague came back to haunt me. "When you have ADD, it can bring out the worst responses in people." My wife was sympathetic, and after hearing that I had lost my job, my friends and family offered support and showed compassion. I became depressed.

One must be cognizant of the frequency of incidences of depression among individuals with ADD. When you live in a world where you can never get on top of your work, and you are formally criticized for falling behind, depression is inevitable. Losing a job is always a blow to self-esteem. Like others who lose their job, I began to question my worth as a husband and a provider. It would take me several months before I was able to find another job.

Not wanting to assume full responsibility, I continued to place blame on the agency from which I was terminated. I collected unemployment until I could find another job. I had thought about going into private practice, and subsequently found a psychiatrist who was willing to let me join his practice. This psychiatrist primarily focused on medication management. The *trickle-down* effect would result in my receiving a handful of referrals. My responsibility would then be to provide individual and family therapy. The referrals were few and far between but they were enough to keep me afloat. The psychiatrist was instrumental in helping me secure full-time work. He contracted with a day treatment program and I was then hired to provide the individual and group therapy for that program.

The program director was my immediate supervisor. She was an RN and had worked in the nursing field for many decades. Coming from a hospital setting, she was used to everything being done "STAT," instantly. (Can you see where this is going?) She did not believe in explaining something more than one time. After one explanation, the worker was expected to appropriately respond to the work environment. I, of course, was not known for my ability to react quickly to environmental cues. Recognizing the subtle nuances of each and every patient was not my strong point. The write-ups began almost immediately. She did not hold back her feelings and was very blunt regarding her opinion of me. I often heard the complaint, "You should know what to do!" I would have to object.

One of the biggest fallacies regarding communication is the belief that an individual should inherently "know" what to do. A person cannot *know* something unless he has been taught. An individual cannot read another person's thoughts. I recall a wife, while in family therapy, telling her husband, "If you loved me, then you'd know what I was thinking." "Hold on a minute," I interjected. "I was unaware that your husband has psychic abilities." People unfairly place this presumptuous burden on others. This is especially unfair to individuals with ADD. Use clear, concise, and explicit instructions regarding what it is that you want the individual to do or say. You have to spell it out. ADD does not provide the luxury of having keen insight into new and unfamiliar situations. I asked this supervisor to be more specific about what it was that she wanted me to do. She did not feel that it was her responsibility to explain. She said, "You'll have to figure it out." Without specific examples, how was I going to do that? I never fully understood this kind of tacit communication. Say what you mean and mean what you say. That's how I was taught to communicate.

As with previous supervisors, I received several character assassinations and condemnations before finally being terminated. On the day I was terminated, my supervisor, using her brilliant observational skills, said, "You look depressed." I had to bite my tongue. I had worked there less than eight months. *Strike three.*

Each termination became more difficult to bear, and with each termination, I had become more defensive. The idea of receiving constructive criticism was frightening. In my world, being criticized always resulted in termination. I was building a wall of protection. I also couldn't bear having to face my wife. She was patient and understanding, but how much longer would she tolerate a husband who couldn't keep a job. This termination came at the worst possible time. My wife and I had just begun a series of costly fertility procedures. We wanted to have a family but would need assisted reproductive procedures to do so. My parents wisely gave my wife a book about adult ADD.

It was one of the few adult ADD books in existence at that time. Around our home, ADD was a sensitive topic. I didn't like to discuss it.

This last job that I had lost was different from others. For the first time, I hadn't been fired for failing to complete paperwork; I was fired for being clueless. Knowing that this was the reason behind my termination, I was awakened to the reality of the breadth and scope of my disorder. It was a harsh reality. I didn't want to admit my limitations. The denial persisted.

Shortly after being fired, I encountered a managed care agency that was looking to contract with private practitioners. I was hired and given an office and a desk. Much to my delight, my scheduling book began to fill with appointments. By listing myself in the on-call rotation, I was able to pick up additional income. I was beginning to make good money. I also kept office hours at the same practice where I worked for the psychiatrist. The paperwork was significantly less challenging; however, procrastination never left my side. The managed care agency eventually closed, but I would be allowed to keep all of my clients and continue in private practice.

After a couple of years had passed, many of the insurance companies terminated their contracts with the various health network providers. As this happened, I lost much of my clientele and had to look for full-time work. A colleague referred me to an agency that provided in-home psychiatric assessments for the elderly. I was hired on the spot. Within a week, I was swamped with referrals. There were numerous forms to complete and protocols that I would have to learn. Good organizational skills would be necessary. After completing my second week of employment, I was called into the director's office. She said, "You're not what we had hoped for. We're letting you go."

Benched!

CHAPTER EIGHT

Cruel Irony

Ironically, the very same profession that I had embraced in the context of wanting to help and advocate for others would be the least tolerant of my disorder. At every turn, my own field of discipline would reject me. My purpose here is not to be cynical, but to make the reader aware of the misperceptions that continue to exist regarding ADD adults. This will become evident as I explain what happened next.

As luck would have it, I was hired as a therapist in a neighboring community. This mental health center was owned and operated under the auspices of a hospital. In addition to providing therapy, I would also be required to participate in on-call rotations in the emergency room, where I would be asked to perform psychiatric assessments. Sometimes I would be paged at 2:00 a.m., and would then have to commute to the ER, a forty-five-minute drive. All the basic ingredients existed that, when combined, would create a stressful job.

For the first year, I managed to juggle an ever-changing caseload. All the staff members were provided with Dictaphones, thus eliminating the time-consuming task of having to write lengthy assessments. Regardless, there were numerous other forms and documents that required meticulous documentation skills. Attention to detail would be essential in order to successfully manage a large caseload. Over time, my caseload doubled in size. My office housed volumes of ominous charts, looking more like a library than a therapist's office.

My mathematical learning disability and problems with spatial relations made an encore performance. All of the therapist's work activities had to be coded on a daily activity log. This activity log contained numerous lines and columns. Special numeric codes signified and indicated in what type of activity the therapist had engaged. The numbers would then be tallied, calculating the sum total. I could never correctly add my numbers. More often than not, I would put the numbers in the wrong columns. These activity logs were constantly returned to me. They were marked in red pen indicating the need for correction. Sometimes they would be returned a second and third time. This caught my supervisor's attention.

Thorough chart reviews were conducted on a regular basis. A utilization review form would be given to the therapist, notifying the worker of any deficiencies found in his chart. I would receive pages of these utilization review forms. I couldn't keep up with them. I was falling further behind in my work. Having ADD at a job that required superfluous amounts of paperwork was a no-win situation. The inevitable write-up would once again rear its ugly head. My supervisor was critical of my productivity numbers. I protested, stating that numbers and statistics were quantitative and a poor indicator of the quality therapy being provided to the clients. The supervisor conceded that my clinical skills were sharp and that I was clinically sound; however, that didn't matter because this agency's standard of measure was numerical.

Several months after that conversation, I would be given a second write-up. In tears, I told my wife that I was facing another termination. In fact, my supervisor told me that a second write-up was like the final nail in the coffin and that I would eventually be let go. I asked the supervisor if he would reconsider and withdraw the write-up. He declined.

I was depressed, and I could no longer deny the fact that I had ADD. My parents, sisters, and my wife were insistent that I fight for my job and claim rights as an employee with a disability. "What rights?" I asked. My family began searching the Internet and found websites that offered information about the Americans With Disability Act and ADD. I spoke with the hospital's director of risk management, asking her if there was anything that I could do to save my job. She was an attorney and was instrumental in dissuading the hospital from immediately terminating me. At first, my supervisor expressed a desire to work with me and seemed genuine in his offer of wanting to "understand your problem." At his request, he met with my parents to gather more information about my history of ADD and learning disabilities. When Human Resources became involved, that would all change.

Someone in Human Resources had decided that my claim of a disability was absurd. I was confronted about my claim. By law, the hospital had a right to request documentation substantiating my disability. My parents had offered my supervisor a stack of historical data, including copies of my IEP, statements from my physician, and other pertinent information. He initially declined. When given this documentation, Human Resources responded by stating, "This doesn't tell us anything. It doesn't prove that you have a disability." I contacted Arizona State University's Disabled Student Services and requested that they send a letter to the hospital verifying my eligibility. Human Resources received the letter and responded: "Although your letter states that you received services through Disabled Student Services, nowhere does it state that you actually have a disability." I met with both the president and vice president of Human Resources. They made it abundantly clear that they wanted a note from my physician confirming the existence of a disability. I argued that my current physician would have no knowledge of my learning disability. I further explained that a physician would not possess the testing instruments and diagnostic tools necessary to diagnose a learning disability.

My supervisor's tone began to parallel that of Human Resource's. He became a skeptic. In a formal reprimand, he described the problematic behaviors relevant to my functioning in the work environment. He said, "Ian does not complete his work in a timely manner. He can often be seen talking to peers and pacing the halls. He fails to follow through with assigned tasks. He forgets to complete tasks. He has fallen behind in his work. Even when given a list of missing assignments, Ian fails to complete the work." This supervisor had just described ADD! His intolerance grew. He began to scrutinize my work. If I asked for clarification regarding a task, he would respond by stating, "I've already explained how to do that." Forgetfulness is a symptom common to ADD adults and children. However, in respect to forgetfulness, a common theme existed: *"If I've already explained it once, then you're not allowed to forget."* Forgetfulness is an unpardonable sin.

Stress and anxiety can increase chronic forgetfulness. As a mental health therapist, I knew that one of the symptoms of anxiety is having difficulty remembering tasks and assignments. Anyone who has ever been in a stressful situation can remember a time when he or she has completely overlooked something important. With ADD, increased anxiety further compounds forgetfulness. The more overwhelmed I became, the more I would forget.

My supervisor, taking advantage of my forgetfulness, would document my every mistake. My anxiety increased, and a vicious cycle ensued. Anxiety is almost always accompanied by depression. I was slipping back into feelings of hopelessness and helplessness. This becomes a dangerous situation because depression is the precursor to "shutting down."

For an individual with ADD, the "shutdown mode" represents the lowest possible level of functioning. When a person reaches that stage, he is simply taking up space. On more than one occasion I have been in that mode. When I went to work, I would be lucky if I could complete one simple task before the day's end. Although there is a depressive factor at play, this is different from suffering from a major depressive episode. The two disorders can at times overlap. However, with clinical depression, concentration and attention span can return to a normal level of functioning, absent of any ADD symptomatalogy. Anxiety and depression exacerbate already existing ADD symptoms. Nevertheless, my family urged me to continue fighting for my job. My wife explained that once and for all I needed to stand up for myself.

I sought updated testing from the college where my father was employed. When I was a child, the college's Learning Resource Center had tested me. Almost twenty years later, they would test me again. A learning disability specialist who contracted with not only the college, but also the public school district tested me. Using the most widely accepted diagnostic tools, his test results were recognized as credible. The testing conclusively established the existence of a learning disability, in addition to the presence of ADD. The hospital immediately questioned the wording of the test results. It now became a semantics issue. "The results still don't clearly state that you have ADD or a disability, and the testing doesn't tell us what you don't have." They also questioned the integrity of the results because the individual who conducted the testing was contracted with the same college where my father had been employed. It was ludicrous. With my father uninvolved, I had independently requested the testing. I made all the necessary contacts and told no one why I needed the testing. Neither my father nor the examiner knew each other. It was completely objective. The hospital raised questions regarding statistical terminology such as "points to" and "indicates," arguing the absence of 100 percent certainty. Keep in mind that none of the Human Resource's staff had any formal training in the interpretation of LD testing, or its common jargon. They wanted to split hairs. I was told, "If you can read then you can't possibly have a learning disability"—another absurd assumption.

For the vice president of Human Resources, the conflict became personal. On more than one occasion, he had bawled me out for questioning his knowledge. I had dared to question it again. Reasoning, diplomacy, and compassion had now been replaced by pride, ego, and arrogance. My immediate supervisor began to institute the use of abject humiliation. I was denied the right to attend continuing education conferences necessary to maintain my clinical license. I requested that I be given several days to catch up on paperwork. This request was denied. Instead, I was mandated to take several days off, but I still continued to come into the office to complete work. I was told that I would not receive regular pay for those weekdays that I had worked, and the money I received would be deducted from my vacation pay. I was being punished—an ignominious corrective action.

Like many people with ADD, it would take me twice as long to catch up on overdue paperwork. By my having to document the completion of every task and form, every minute of my working day became scrutinized. At the end of the day, my supervisor would declare, "Is that all that you've done today? Anybody could have done more than that!" I now was being threatened with termination on a fairly regular basis. I had finally had enough, and for the first time in my life, I advocated for myself. At a significant financial cost, I retained an attorney. He advised me as to the next path to take.

A colleague directed me to a well-respected and professionally recognized expert in adult ADD. I would have to travel to the Chicago suburbs for further testing. I presented this psychologist with all of my historical data, including the most recent testing that had been rejected by Human Resources. After reviewing all of the data, the psychologist expressed disbelief at the hospital's unwillingness to yield. I was retested. The results were compelling. The psychologist wrote a lengthy synopsis of the assessment. He stated that I definitively and unequivocally had "severe ADD, in addition to a learning disability." He would use the term "severe" several times throughout his report. He noted that on two of the conducted tests, my short-term memory recall fell within the 13th percentile. On another memory test I had scored as low as the 1st percentile, an ADD red flag. After discussing my test results, I felt a sense of relief. I now had to finally accept the extent of my disability. I could no longer deceive myself, not even in part. It was a sobering moment.

My supervisor had said to me, "I don't believe that you have ADD," but he didn't stop there. In response to the LCSW that I had worked so hard to achieve, he stated, "I don't even think of you as an LCSW." Children can be cruel; adults can be crueler. People with ADD must realize that just because an individual offers an insipid opinion about whether or not you have ADD, this does not negate the validity of the disorder's existence. It is only one person's feelings and is not based on any objective observation or experience. ADD is inherently different from other disabilities. When a disability such as ADD is not obvious or easily perceived, many will tend to reject what they can't see or understand.

The Human Resources Department had received the test results. A formal letter would clarify their position. Almost immediately, the hospital would use the phrase "and without acknowledging that you have a 'disability,' we will look at several recommendations concerning your 'condition.'" These people had been speaking with their attorney. They knew that if they admitted that I had a disability, then they would fall under the auspices of several legal mandates. They weren't about to do that. From then on, in reference to ADD, my supervisor and members of Human

Resources would only use the term "condition." I began asking myself, "What kind of a mental health agency/hospital organization would be so obtuse and, go to such great lengths to do everything possible not to recognize or provide accommodations for a disabled employee?" Many professionals with whom I worked began to question the work ethics of such an organization. This employer was interested in termination not accommodation.

The hospital would eventually receive a letter from my attorney. My supervisor replied, "So what, a lot of people have ADD. That doesn't mean anything." He then began to make ADD analogous to prostate cancer. "It's like saying 'I *had* prostate cancer, but now I don't,'" he explained. He was trying to tell me that ADD could be cured. Was this guy for real? He was the clinical director of a large mental health center and also held a clinical license in social work. Surely he knew that ADD and learning disabilities aren't simply *cured*. I requested the assistance of a job coach, specializing in adult ADD. This request was rejected. Instead, I received another letter from the vice president of Human Resources. Instead of recognizing the concerns raised by my attorney, he went into a lengthy discourse about what accommodations "we don't have to provide." He boastfully explained that I had limited legal rights. Again, by retaining an attorney, I had threatened his ego, an ego that by all rights needed its own zip code. The employee's welfare was not this employer's concern.

I would receive only one reasonable accommodation, a "peer mentor." This co-worker's responsibility was to check my work and tell me what I hadn't completed. Didn't I already have a supervisor who did that? These people had dug in their heels, and their intransigence was obvious. I began looking elsewhere for employment, but the job market was tight. With the exception of moving from Utah back to Illinois, I had never quit a job. Quitting my job would be financial suicide. With no other employment prospects, I would stay right where I was.

The hospital was in a precarious predicament. If they fired me without making reasonable accommodations, they could be left open to a lawsuit. If they wanted me gone, they would have to find another way. Late one evening, a colleague approached me and asked me if I would conduct a crisis assessment for a client. I declined. I explained that I was tired, hungry, and was leaving for my dinner break. I further explained that my supervisor, on several occasions, had reprimanded me for rendering assistance to the Crisis Department. He made it perfectly clear that my main priority should be the completion of my paperwork. It was not uncommon for therapists to be sent to the ER to assist in the backlog of psychiatric consults. I had done this many times, but now had been told to stay away from the Crisis Department.

About a week later, I was called into the Human Resources office. There, the president of Human Resources and my supervisor met me. An interrogation ensued. I was asked specifically what I was doing on the evening November 21, 2000, at or around 4:45 p.m. Not knowing exactly where they were going with this question, I responded, "How am I supposed to remember what I was doing eight days ago?" "You would remember if you had refused to treat a patient," was the reply. And there it was. I was being accused of refusing to treat a patient. Their version of events was much different from what had happened. The hospital would claim that a supervisor, not a colleague, had directed me to treat a patient and that I had adamantly disobeyed the directive. I corrected the hospital, explaining that my supervisor had told me not to assist the Crisis Department, and that it was a colleague, not a supervisor, who had requested my assistance. It was a "double bind," I argued, and I further explained that when I left for dinner, another worker was assessing the client. "Well, we'll look into the facts," was the response. I was suspended with pay.

A week later I would return to the hospital. "After conducting a thorough investigation," it was explained to me that evidence "from multiple witnesses," definitively concluded that I had lied about the event in question. I asked, "Who are these witnesses and what did they say?" I was given no response. These people were ruthless and diabolical. I was fired on the spot. *Ejected from the game!*

I had been fired again. I had mixed feelings about the efficacy of my attorney. For eight months he was able to stave off my termination. Sure, pursuing legal retaliation was an option, but at great risk. To date, no strong ADD case law or precedent exists where the resulting outcome has been favorable. There were no guarantees as to the outcome of a trial. Also, it would cost me thousands of dollars to pursue such action. Even if the Equal Employment Opportunity Commission (EEOC) and the Department of Human Rights agreed with my complaint, it would all come down to money. It wasn't worth it. After filing complaints with both the EEOC and the Department of Human Rights, I was happy to finally be rid of the hospital and its minions.

Within two weeks of being fired, I was offered another job. An agency had responded to a resume that I had sent several months before. I went to the interview expecting to be hired as a therapist. When I returned home, I received a phone call from the interviewer. I was being offered the position of clinical director. I had always been clinically sound and on many occasions had been commended for my clinical competency. I then took the biggest gamble of my life. I explained that I had been fired from previous employers and that I had both ADD and a learning disability. This disclosure would pay off. I was given "reasonable accommodations" and was told that the position for which I was being hired would not require much paperwork.

The hospital, of course, would fight my unemployment benefits. In a scathing letter from the Department of Employment Security, the hospital was admonished for not providing any evidence, including witnesses, to substantiate their claim of "willful misconduct." I think that they were a little frightened by the letter because, to no avail, they would proceed to file two more appeals, losing each one.

What had I gained from this experience? I definitely had to reevaluate my ADD. I decided that I would be frank and forthright with all of my supervisors. It was time for me to start taking control and assume full responsibility for my disorder. My parents had always cautioned me against using ADD as an excuse. Until I was on the verge of losing my last job, I had never *told* anyone that I even had ADD. I would now explain my disorder, being careful not to offer the explanation as an excuse. I devised a completely new game plan.

At present, I continue working in clinical management. My success, however, came with a price. I had to be fired five times before the proverbial light bulb above my head finally turned on. Call me a slow learner. But my story does not end here; it begins. In the following section, I will explain how I took the next step from understanding why I was fired to preventing it from happening again.

PART IV

Solutions

CHAPTER NINE

Devising a Game Plan

The comments in this section are directed at not only those individuals who have ADD but also the people with whom they associate. Again, I draw on my own experiences to further illustrate pragmatic solutions. As you read this section, it is important to note that it is your choice as to which management techniques you choose to utilize. Be open-minded and willing to explore and examine different points of view and perceptions regarding ADD. Think for yourself. As others could not think for me, I had to assume responsibility in managing this disorder.

Think about managing ADD as though it were a sport. As with all sports, you must first learn the rules. You will also need a coach. A coach is someone who can teach you how to improve your game and advise you on calling plays. As do gymnasts, you will need a "spotter," in case you should fall. Development and improvement of skills comes with practice. A coach or a spotter can review your performance and make suggestions for improvement.

Procrastination is the first obstacle that must be confronted. Often referred to as "the thief of time," procrastination stalks ADD people like a lion stalks its prey. Unlike *The Terminator*, who says, "I'll be back,"

The Procrastinator says, "I'll be back—eventually." The feelings and desire to put things off will not magically disappear. While spending hundreds of dollars, many people attend seminars that offer the promise of complete freedom from procrastination. This is not realistic. Procrastination is an endogenous function of ADD. It doesn't go away. Since you're not going to *get over* procrastination; the trick is learning how to *get around* procrastination. When I go to work, I focus on one or two main objectives. All other tasks and assignments are secondary to that objective. For example, one of my objectives might be to complete a report and then FAX it to my supervisor. This means that I have chosen that task as the most urgent task to be completed. Everything else is considered of less importance. I may jump from one task to another, but that's okay as long as I keep coming back to the main objective. Sometimes looking at the big picture is the wrong approach. Don't go to work thinking about *all the things* that I have to do today. Go to work thinking about the *most important* thing I have to do today. The rest will fall into place.

When working, I easily grow restless. Rather than staying in one place, throughout the day, I will often work from more than one location within the office. This allows me the freedom to change scenery and burn off pent-up energy. I am a chronic pacer. Supervisors notice pacers. A better approach would be to leave for a bathroom break or take a short walk around the building. Some people are not provided with that luxury. If such is the case, ask your supervisor if might be possible to work from a different location or work at a different machine. This is especially helpful for individuals who work in a shop or on an assembly line.

Always carry a pen and paper. Become comfortable with the idea of always having a note pad at your side. Let it be your constant companion. Write everything down. Don't be afraid to ask others to assist. Yes, it is important to function independently, but if someone is willing to jot down a few notes in your behalf, then don't refuse such a resource. When consulting with co-workers, I have noticed some of my colleagues are acutely aware of my memory limitations. As if by instinct, they ask, "Do you want me to write that down for you?" My supervisor will occasionally offer to document a task list, especially during impromptu conferences where many tasks are assigned. Again, the primary responsibility rests upon the ADD individual. You must make taking notes a habit. Another effective organizational tool is a Palm Pilot. A Dictaphone can quickly store verbal reminders. Record, rewind, and press "Play."

The best defense is a good offense. That means learning to recognize your defensive behaviors. Defensiveness breeds negative responses from others. Defensive statements are easy to spot. If you find yourself always having to offer an explanation for your actions, then you're being defensive. If you are constantly making excuses, then you're being defensive. Do you interpret all constructive feedback as criticism? Do you get anxious during routine meetings with your supervisor? When discussing work issues, it is important to pay attention to your verbal and nonverbal responses. Supervisors have to do their job, and that means that they will review, supervise, and critique your work. If a supervisor offers a suggestion, your response should be, "That's a good idea and I'll give it a try." If asked for an explanation of a task, calmly respond, offering only the facts. Maintain a neutral tone. Take deep breaths and relax. Your supervisor's duties should not be personalized. It is unpleasant to work with an individual who personalizes everything. Accept feedback and learn from it. Listen to suggestions and take advice. Change is good, so don't be afraid to change how you approach working with others.

For the longest time, I was unaware of my defensiveness and, on more than one occasion, I'm certain that this defensiveness cost me my job. An example of this defensiveness would occur when a supervisor would ask me a simple, non-judgmental question. Instead of giving a simple response, my responses were abrupt. I was only being asked to respond to a simple question, but I felt like I was on trial for witchcraft. Today, I've learned when to keep my mouth shut (most of the time). When an individual is angry, that is when he should be the most vigilant in maintaining silence. Reactive responses are never healthy and almost always result in a negative outcome. Persons with ADD must learn this concept as though their very lives depend on it. During my late teens, I became a big *Star Trek* fan. Mr. Spock was the character I most admired. He embodied everything

I wanted to be. Although he was fictional, I envied his ability to calmly handle any situation, devoid of emotionally filled responses. During my career, when asked to testify in court, I would often go into what I liked to refer as "Vulcan mode." I knew that when I was on the stand testifying, I could not afford to give ADD-saturated answers. Eliminating these defensive responses takes practice and patience.

CHAPTER TEN

Gaining Insight—The Big Risk

To gain insight into one's behavior, one must be willing to accept constructive feedback.

This becomes a big risk because you must be willing to acknowledge personal weakness and faults. Your self-esteem must be strong enough to withstand forthright honesty and frankness. Asking for feedback leaves open the vulnerable spots in each of us; however, it is worth undertaking such a risk. Let others be your eyes and ears. Ask for the opinions of others. Earlier, we discussed the importance of having a coach or a spotter. Let that person(s) provide you with life-giving insight.

Take note of how people respond to your comments, gestures, and tone. By the time I entered my early teens, I began to notice that my incessant talking elicited a negative response from others. Over time, I realized that I needed to listen more and talk less. As a therapist, when speaking with my clients, I *had* to develop listening skills and force myself to maintain eye contact. I soon discovered that my relationships were far more meaningful when mutual reciprocity existed. People with ADD must learn that life is a give-and-take relationship. After years of working as a therapist, I have learned that the most self-absorbed and egocentric people are the ones who have no insight.

Misunderstanding the governing principles of human relations, these people become so wrapped up in their own personal problems and disorders that their life becomes a world of wasted opportunities. ADD creates a life with distractions, but that doesn't mean that you have to be distracted from life.

Being a therapist would dramatically improve my writing skills. After conducting hundreds of assessments, I learned to write quickly and efficiently. I had completely overcome that childhood struggle. I also gained the insight of knowing that weaknesses could later become strengths. Although I write well, I inadvertently omit words. My learning disability has largely contributed to this problem. I can proofread my written work, honestly believing that every word is present and accounted for. More often than not, several words *are* missing. My brain doesn't seem to know the difference. Knowing that this is a weakness, I always ask someone else to proofread my work.

Bank tellers cringe when they see me walk in the door. I am, for all practical purposes, a bank teller's worst nightmare. Because I have a mathematical learning disability, I always have to have others check my work. Calculators are helpful, but my wife claims that I am the only person she has ever known who, when using a calculator, actually makes more mistakes than if I had not used a calculator. Wisely, I have my wife balance our checking account and handle most of our bills. When I pay in cash, I always make sure to ask the cashier to count my money. "Believe me," I exclaim, "it's to your advantage."

The constant distraction of extraneous noise can be overwhelming. When at work, I am involved in numerous consultations. While other staff may be able to simultaneously speak and block out background noise, I cannot. I have learned to close doors. Like many people with ADD, I have problems with auditory discrimination. Noises coming from different locations are all heard at the same level. It's annoying but this is my reality. Sometimes I move to a quieter location. I am comfortable asking co-workers and supervisors to close doors or meet with me in an alternate location. If you have ADD but don't make a habit of doing this, then you are allowing yourself to continue being a victim. Why subject yourself to that kind of misery, when simple communication can offer a simple solution?

It is difficult to hide symptoms of distraction. I have found that people can easily recognize when a person is having difficulty focusing. Don't pretend to pay attention. While in session with clients, I have often asked the client if it would be okay for me to close a window to limit distractions. People understand, and you may discover that they are being distracted by some of the very same things that are distracting you.

People are quick to notice avoidant behavior. This can become a problem because ADD is wrought with the drive and temptation to steer far from tasks requiring sustained mental or physical effort. Everyone knows the resentful feelings that are directed toward the employee who "does nothing." While everyone else is putting forth his best effort, there's always that *one* employee who gets out of having to do his work. Don't be *that* employee.

ADD people thrive in a neat, clean, and organized environment. Ironically, they are ill equipped to structure that very environment where they are most likely to thrive. For example, I hate clutter. The more clutter, the more I become frustrated. More often than not, though, I am usually the author of that clutter. In chapter one, I discussed the pediatrician who advised my parents to remove all excess stimuli from my bedroom. He provided invaluable advice—*less is more*. Where there is less clutter, there is more freedom from distraction. This holds true not only for children but also for adults. When my office or home is free from debris, I feel relaxed compared to the distraction and accompanying anxiety I feel when working or living in a messy place. I have often instructed parents to assist their ADD child in cleaning his room. "Don't wait for the child to do it or it's never going to happen," I explain. Clean both your home and work environment. Get that monkey off your back. This allows both ADD children and adults to start with a fresh, clean slate. All of us have experienced the feelings of relief associated with having finally cleaned a deplorable room. It's a good feeling.

Another problem with clutter is that it creates the perfect environment for misplacing items; therefore, couch gnomes cannot be blamed for lost keys. I walk items around my home. I put them down, walk away and then forget where I last placed them. At one time or another, all of us have done this, but with ADD children and adults, the problem is far more extensive and pervasive. Misplacing items is directly tied to short-term memory impairment. One way of negotiating this problem is to make a list of the most commonly misplaced items. After determining which items are frequently misplaced, then make a determination as to which items are the *most critical.* If lost, which items are the most necessary to your existence? Keys should be one of the first things that come to mind. For others, cell phone, purse, wallet, jewelry, pager, glasses, money, notes, bills, etc., are essential items. Put them in the same place every time. Do not waiver from this habit. Repetition creates memory. Routine and consistency reinforce memory. Every night, I always put my glasses, pager, wallet, wedding band, and pen in the same location. This technique has significantly reduced the frequency of my misplacing items.

Missing the obvious is one of the ADD symptoms for which I am best known. I have the ability to overlook an item that is right in front of my face. I am notorious for accusing my wife of not having bought any butter from the store. This accusation is usually made as I peer into the refrigerator, staring directly at the butter. Another form of *missing the obvious* is not recognizing when someone needs help or assistance. It took me years to recognize situations in which someone might need assistance, and then learn to render that assistance. For example, when a person was in the middle of completing a house chore, yard work, cooking a meal, or cleaning up after an activity, I would speak with that person completely oblivious to the idea that perhaps he or she might need some help. Play it safe; always ask others if they need assistance. Even more importantly, always ask, "Is there anything that I can do for you?"

For me maps are like geometric equations. The numerous lines, crossing patterns, and grids can be confusing. This is especially true when viewing a large city map. The general rule has always been to provide ADD persons with no more than one or two directions at a time. However, in situations involving travel, the use of multiple directions cannot be avoided. If such is the case, make the explanation of how to get there a visual experience. The use of a highlighted marker can illuminate the path from start to finish, similar to tracing a pencil through a maze. Always ask for landmarks or other visual points of reference, so that you are not relying solely upon street names. Some of my greatest moments of frustration have occurred when I have been lost, driving in circles, having lost all bearings. A cell phone is a wonderful tool if one is lost. The one on the other end of the line can provide visual cues and verbal prompts, thus assisting you to your final destination.

To gain insight into the disorder, you must be aware of some of the ADD problem areas that have been discussed. More importantly, when appropriate, you need to make others aware of some of your problem areas. This does not mean that you have to publicly announce your disorder, like the man in the television commercial who tells everyone that he has lowered his cholesterol. Your ADD and learning disabilities are on a *need-to- know* basis. It is a personal choice as to whether or not you share the specifics of your disorder with others. It *is* a risk, and like all risks there are no guarantees as to how others will respond to your disclosure. Most people have heard the term "ADD" but most are unfamiliar with specifics of this disorder in adults. Many are misinformed or have preconceived notions about people with this disorder. Educate. Teach others what you know.

CHAPTER ELEVEN

Taking It Up a Notch

Watching myself on video is one of the most enlightening experiences I have ever had. I was able to view myself in the same way others see me. I truly have ADD. My restlessness is shockingly apparent. I drum my hands and fingers on everything. I *know* that I do this, but until I actually saw myself in action, I was unaware of how noticeable it was. It was like watching a Buddy Rich concert. In fact, during meetings, staff members have often asked me to stop drumming my fingers. Watching myself fidget and repeatedly shift positions was also alarming. It wouldn't take a genius to figure out who in the room has ADD; like the *Sesame Street* song says, "One of these things is not like the other." Two years ago, I was a guest on a local TV show. This station produced a community awareness show that aired on Sunday mornings. I was asked to discuss the specific mission of the agency at which I was employed, and to comment on the clinical implications of children in foster care. Despite knowing how horribly restless I appear when on TV, I still accepted the challenge. I practiced sitting still. I literally sat on my hands in effort to stop myself from drumming or shifting. This time, instead of looking like a puppy on speed, I looked like a stiff board. People who saw the TV show said, "You weren't very animated." I would take that as a compliment. From that experience, I learned that I *could* control my excessive body movement.

The desire for insight must supersede the fear of criticism. Get in the habit of asking the questions "Did I sound defensive?" "How did that sound?" and "Did I seem restless?" Become comfortable in intentionally asking others to identify your oversights. Sometimes, when asked to go get a specific item, I am often unable to locate the item. Rather than saying, "I couldn't find it," I often request that someone else "double-check, because sometimes I miss things." I tell the truth. Don't hide the truth or pretend that nothing is wrong. Everyone has personal deficits. Know your deficits. Be honest with yourself and with others. If you don't remember a specific conversation with a co-worker or a supervisor's directive, then say, "I'm sorry, I don't remember that discussion." Because this forgetfulness does not excuse you from responsibility, your apology should also include a commitment to do a better job at keeping track of future information. Remember, just because you don't remember a specific conversation or event, that doesn't mean that it didn't happen. Many arguments occur as a result of someone stubbornly holding to the belief that the other person is in the wrong. If you forget to complete a task, then say, "I'm sorry, that's my fault; I forgot to do it." If you start to see a pattern of forgetfulness around a specific event or task, then it's time to develop a new, preventative strategy.

Accept the inevitably that you will have bad ADD days, just as you will have good ADD days. On a bad ADD day, I forget everything. I feel a loss of control. I often feel overwhelmed. I am anxious. When such is the case, I have to rely upon some of the previously discussed coping strategies. Sometimes I need to let those around me know that it's going to be "one of those days." If I have a good day, I make sure that I give myself credit by acknowledging my accomplishments and recognizing improvement and progress. Receiving occasional praise and recognition is important for those of us with ADD.

The request for feedback should be a continuous, ongoing process. It's the only way that you're going to learn how to recognize and modify your ADD behaviors. Think of it as a means to an end. Accept constructive feedback. Rise to the challenge, and be reminded that you are of importance and self-worth. Though limitations accompany ADD, do not place unnecessary limitations upon yourself.

Better than anyone else, sometimes you know the best solutions to your problems. I have worked with many different supervisors. At one time or another, each of them has offered what they believed to be a quick and simple solution to my ADD symptoms. Their solution is usually worded something like, "All you have to do is…." This type of concrete and simplistic thinking is a manifestation of society's continued ignorance of ADD and an unwillingness to go beyond the concept that "one simplistic solution fits all." Supervisors have reprimanded me for not employing their recommended interventions. This has occurred even after I have explained that although their method of tracking information may seem effective, another tracking method would be more appropriate for one with my disorder. Be prepared to defend those interventions that you know to be effective. This does not mean that you should be close-minded to other possibilities, but it does mean that you should not be forced into utilizing a technique that does not work for you.

CHAPTER TWELVE

Have a Sense of Humor

I use humor as a stress reliever and also because I believe that people should enjoy life. Many people take *life* and *themselves* too seriously. Something is inherently wrong when we are unable to relax and have a good laugh about something funny that has just happened. Being able to put a humorous twist on a stressful situation requires talent and creativity. I realize that there are many people who simply don't know how to look for or appreciate the appropriate use of humor. That is most unfortunate. Those people are missing golden opportunities, through the use of humor, to further enhance and develop their relationships with others.

When you have ADD or you work with persons with ADD, you *have* to have a sense of humor. I have had to learn to laugh at myself. Sometimes we make mistakes that *are* funny. When working or living with ADD individuals, be careful that you first gage the person's ability to handle humor, so that they do not perceive your humor as a criticism. Some ADD people (and such was the case with me) do not always recognize a joke. Teach them that sometimes it's okay to laugh at oneself. The message should be clear—*lighten up!*

Now, a word of caution regarding humor. When you have ADD, sometimes the spontaneity of a humorous comment can be inappropriate. There is a time and a place for everything and it takes wisdom to know the difference. Childish, impulsive pranks can have negative repercussions. I have seen many ADD people exercise poor judgment through such impulsive humor. In the sixth grade, on a field trip to the Museum of Natural History in Chicago, Illinois, my friend Steve and I thought it might be amusing to break a few rules. The sign posted outside the King Tut exhibit explicitly forbid the use of flash photography. In fact, cameras were forbidden inside the exhibit. All cameras had to be turned in prior to viewing the archeological collection. Partly on my insistence, Steve and I decided that would it be "real cool" if we took our own picture of the famous Golden Mask. We smuggled a camera into the exhibit. That day Steve and I learned that when you take a flash picture of an object that is not allowed to be photographed, you draw unwanted attention. Fortunately, nothing serious happened other than a harsh reprimand from our sixth-grade teacher, who was relieved to have averted an international incident.

CHAPTER THIRTEEN

Interpreting and Accepting ADD

The comments of this chapter are directed at those who employ or live with an ADD individual. When interacting with a person with ADD, you may experience frequent frustration. Please understand that the ADD individual is experiencing that same frustration, only two-fold. Not only is he struggling to organize and remember his daily tasks, but he is also trying to balance and manage your frustration with him, of which he is keenly aware.

Don't criticize ADD symptoms. Under no circumstances should you engage in labeling. Those of us with this disorder have already experienced a lifetime of name-calling and related criticisms. We don't need to be reminded of that which we already know. Sadly, I have seen many adults who, after losing their job, have then had to withstand the wrath of an unforgiving spouse. I have been fired five times; not once did my wife ever accuse me of being lazy or question my role as a husband and a provider. She knew that I needed support. My parents, likewise, never engaged in such destructive criticism.

Like many people who have worked a long day, after returning home, ADD people need time to relax.

That is not the time to engage them in a lengthy conversation, discuss bills, ask them to take out the trash, or make major life decisions. Let them be. In time, they will come around and be ready to rejoin the family. Spouses and family members should not take this behavior personally. Many people feel that their ADD spouse is rejecting them or doesn't care about their feelings. This is not true. Allow the down time and space that he or she needs. That same respect is due to all persons, regardless of an ADD diagnosis.

Some people personalize situations in which the memory-challenged spouse has forgotten to do something that you have asked. They misinterpret this forgetfulness as a passive-aggressive behavior. When after five requests he still has not taken out the garbage, they are tempted to label their spouse as "lazy." Again, you must separate the individual from the disorder. Rather than complaining about your spouse's weaknesses, try praising and complimenting his strengths.

The creation of an ADD-friendly environment, as previously discussed, can help in assisting your ADD spouse or family member. Verbal prompts and other reminders aid in cuing that individual into remembering tasks. If we are asking for help, those of us with ADD must be willing to accept verbal prompts and not interpret spousal reminders as incessant "nagging." Finding a homeostatic balance between *reminding* and *nagging* takes time and patience. At one time or another, most couples have been ensnared in this dilemma.

There are inherent problems associated with ADD individuals and employment. Most employers would never knowingly hire an employee with ADD. Let's be honest. How many employers, when weighing the qualifications of one applicant against another, are going to say, "You know I really like this candidate, Mr. Jones, but unlike Mr. Smith, who shares the same credentials and work experiences, Mr. Jones has ADD and offers the challenge of low work productivity, procrastination, and chronic forgetfulness. Let's hire him." That just doesn't happen. Most people, if hired, were offered the position because they interviewed well, were a better, qualified candidate, or the employer needed the position filled immediately. They weren't hired for having ADD. Many companies have policies that prevent them from sharing information about previous employees; thus, anyone inquiring about the candidate's work history will only be told their hire date and last date of employment. The law prevents an employer from asking a prospective hire whether or not he has a disability. Finally, most prospective employees would never begin an interview by stating, "I have ADD." The employer won't figure that out until sometime later. Even then, unless trained in social work, education, or psychology, the employer will simply refer to the worker being as lazy and ineffective.

If you have an employee with ADD, you must first come to terms with your own issues regarding this disorder. People, who are viewed as lazy, slow, or ineffective, usually elicit negative feelings. This is especially true when the ADD employee reminds the employer of someone from his own past, or even himself. Freud called this process *transference*. Some employers resent the fact that they unknowingly hired a person with ADD. Most companies are only interested in running their business and cannot be bothered with having to manage an ADD employee. If perceived as the weakest link in the chain, that employee is expendable.

The employer should ask himself if he is willing or able to capitalize on the strengths of the ADD employee. What most employers don't know is that the overwhelming majority of people with ADD are of *above average intelligence*. Many are very creative and possess certain skills and talents. The key to the employee's success is for the employer to identify which of those talents will most benefit the company. ADD people who do thrive in their work environment do so because their idiosyncrasies and talents are an asset to the employer. Everybody wins. Whenever possible, an employer should consider job restructuring or modifying the employee's job description. Remember that even when an employee has been given accommodations, it is reasonable to expect improvement, but it is unreasonable to expect or require the employee to stop having ADD.

Yes, there are legal loopholes and limitations regarding what reasonable accommodations a company is mandated to provide for its ADD employees. This, however, should not deter employees from seeking accommodations or challenging the laws. This issue comes down to only *one* question: is the company interested in *accommodation* or *termination*?

There is a dichotomy in the social work profession. Our profession seeks to employ individuals who are willing to provide treatment and assistance to persons with *problems,* including ADD. However, when the employee has ADD, these rules may change. ADD is then perceived not as a disorder but as a personal weakness. After disclosing my ADD, I have often heard responses like, "Then what are you doing in this profession?" Some disorders, like cerebral palsy, are lifetime conditions. We aren't expecting people with cerebral palsy to outgrow their condition. Why are we asking people with ADD to outgrow this lifetime disorder? Statements like, "Well, you're a professional now and it's time to put that disorder aside," are not only absurd but indicate the alarming degree of ignorance among social work employers. The human service professions will attract employees who are skilled at working with people. Inevitably, some of these genuinely talented and compassionate workers will themselves have ADD. The profession must then decide which approach to take. If ADD employees are pushed out of the profession, then hypocrisy prevails. Superfluous amounts of paperwork, large caseloads, and long work hours all contribute to the ADD employee's demise. Their clients also suffer.

To some, these comments may seem like they are my own personal issues and internalized rhetoric.

That would be a false assumption. In working with ADD adults, I have found that many of them, like me, have had similar, negative work experiences. They make similar observations. They have expressed their feelings of and frustration with having no one in their corner, or when at work, feeling helpless and alone. For them, this is not rhetoric; it *is* reality.

ADD is not just an individual problem; it is also a societal problem. ADD people who cannot hold a job will collect unemployment, a burden passed on to the taxpayer. As previously stated, if placed in the right work environment, most ADD people who are intelligent and professionally skilled will thrive. Society should be flexible and willing to provide "reasonable accommodations" for its ADD employees.

ADD people can change. The change of which I am speaking does not mean that they will no longer have ADD, but people can change their approach to managing the disorder. However, as ADD is lifelong disorder, the process and degree of change is largely dependent on the individual's insight and maturity, as discussed in previous chapters. Do not assume that a twenty-one-year-old ADD adult will behave the same way at age thirty-one. The same is also true of ADD children. Do not become disheartened. When I was fourteen years old, my parents could not have predicted that I would complete a master's degree, obtain a clinical license, and then go on to become the clinical director of an agency. Personal growth may not occur as quickly as you would like. Patience is required.

My ADD and specific learning disability in math are very much alive. I still struggle with procrastination. I like to avoid activities or work that requires sustained mental effort. At work, even with interventions, I will have ADD moments in which I have completely overlooked a task or have forgotten to follow through with an assignment. I still misplace items both at home and at work. I am constantly on guard, apologizing if I inadvertently interrupt someone. I watch carefully for defensive statements and behaviors. I ask my supervisor and co-workers to help me identify when such defensiveness is occurring. If I need help, I ask for it. If I need more time to complete an assignment, I then ask for it. I still stare into the refrigerator, looking for the butter. Some days I become frustrated and get discouraged. My math skills are still that of a fourth-grader's, so I won't be building rockets for NASA.

ADD people should find joy in life. As previously discussed, humor is essential to my existence. I have various hobbies and interests. For me, music is an important outlet. I am a member of a cover band where I play bass guitar and keyboards. My membership in a band came as a result of my constant desire to drum my fingers, now channeled into a healthy activity. I enjoy reading. I used to hate reading. I could never stay with a book long enough to enjoy the plot. Large, thick books intimidated my attention span. I didn't start reading "for fun" until I was thirty-one years old. I have now read dozens of classic literary works. My wife is perplexed. "I don't understand it," she would exclaim. "You hate reading!" People can change. Weaknesses can become strengths.

Notwithstanding the commonalities of ADD, the manifestation of this disorder is unique to each individual. While one person may struggle with fidgeting and restlessness, to another, those same symptoms may not be as problematic. Idiosyncrasies and personality nuances also define the uniqueness of the disorder, i.e., *the symptoms are similar but the people are different*. My life experiences have largely influenced the manifestation of my ADD; however, some of my recommended interventions are applicable regardless of one's life circumstances. As one passes through different phases of life, interventions are modified and revisions made.

HELPFUL SUGGESTIONS AND INSIGHTS
for ADD Adults

1. *Ask for accommodations.* Don't wait until you're in over your head. Your employer can't address your struggles if he or she doesn't know of their existence. You have a legal right to request reasonable accommodations.

2. *Disclose.* As previously discussed, disclosing your ADD involves risk. You may fear rejection or criticism. If you are not sure when it is appropriate to disclose your ADD then consult an objective friend or professional advocate.

3. *Be honest with yourself.* Be willing to admit that you have a problem. This means avoiding denial. Do not fall victim to shame and its accompanying emotions. Don't run from ADD, but instead confront it. Accept your limitations, but recognize your strengths.

4. *Gain insight through feedback.* Ask for feedback. Be willing to have others critique your behaviors and symptoms. Let people know of the symptoms with which you struggle. Don't be defensive when such constructive feedback is offered. Learn from these experiences.

5. *Find a coach.* A close friend, family member, spouse, or employer, all can prompt and encourage you. Find people who are willing to cheer you on and advocate on your behalf. Occasionally, everybody needs a cheering section.

6. *Prioritize and simplify.* Remember, one task at a time, one day at a time. Do not over-schedule or create extra, unnecessary work. Focus on what is *most* important, e.g., paying the bills. (Many ADD people believe that bills pay themselves.) Be on the offense against procrastination.

7. *Have a sense of humor.* Don't be so serious about life that you fail to enjoy it. Learn to laugh at yourself and recognize appropriate use of humor.

8. *Don't lie.* If you forget to complete a task, make a mistake or misplace an item, then tell the truth. Honest people are respected. Lying only complicates the problem.

9. *Engage in stress-relieving activities.* Pursue hobbies and other interests. Eat right and exercise. Take frequent breaks when possible. Allow for downtime. Tell others when you need to have time to yourself. Learn to recognize stress.

10. *Seek legal assistance.* This should always be a last resort. If you truly believe that someone is discriminating against you or is failing to provide reasonable accommodations, then consult an attorney. Make sure that the person with whom you speak specializes in disability and discrimination law. They can advise you on the appropriate use of the EEOC and the Department of Human Rights.

HELPFUL SUGGESTIONS AND INSIGHTS
for Family, Friends, and Employers

1. *Don't criticize.* Criticizing ADD accomplishes nothing. Criticism undermines self-esteem development, resulting in increased defensiveness and feelings of self-doubt. Nobody wins.

2. *Be flexible.* Don't hold on to rigid performance expectations. Be willing to explore various options for managing ADD symptoms. If you employ someone with ADD, allow for reasonable accommodations. Focus on the employer's strengths. Ask the ADD employee what accommodations might work.

3. *Listen.* Like all individuals, people with ADD need to be heard and to feel validated. Offer feedback, but also be open-minded and honestly seek realistic ways to improve the ADD person's overall functioning.

4. *Be realistic.* Remember that ADD and accompanying learning disabilities are a lifetime condition. Don't impose unrealistic expectations. Don't expect them to stop having ADD. They won't *get over* ADD, but together you can create ways to *get around* ADD.

5. *Allow for downtime.* People with ADD take longer to unwind. Permit them to have a period of peace and quite. Likewise, take time out for yourself. You deserve it and you'll need it in long-term association with ADD.

6. *Don't personalize*. Do not interpret ADD behaviors as being passive-aggressive, spiteful, or vindictive. ADD behaviors are the result of a disorder. The symptoms are endogenous to that disorder and are not being directed specifically at you. You do have a right to express your frustrations. Stating, *"When you ... I feel,"* allows for both ownership and validation of feelings, without placing blame.

7. *Seek support*. As a person who lives or works with an ADD individual, sometimes you need support and validation. ADD support groups are not just for people with ADD, but also for the ADD person's parents, family, friends, and co-workers.

8. *Educate yourself.* Knowledge is an effective weapon. Arm yourself with the latest information and techniques on living with ADD. Become familiar with new medications and current research data. Attend trainings.

9. *Give praise*. Everyone needs to feel of worth. When addressing self-esteem, justified compliments are important. Recognition of accomplishments and achievements are paramount. It is important to acknowledge even the smallest milestone.

10. *Be an advocate.* Take on the role of a coach. Offer to be a mentor. Become an educational advocate. Start your own support group. Volunteer your talents and skills. Teach others what you know. People with ADD remember those who advocate on their behalf. Your

community will also benefit from your service, for many who struggle to live with their ADD have talent, skills, and insight to improve the society in which they live

CONCLUSION

Attention Deficit Disorder is a condition that, for many, has disabling symptoms that continue well into adulthood. Although we recognize this disorder in children, as a society we tend to overlook its impact on adults. We falsely believe that the individual will *outgrow* the disorder. Consequently, when confronted with an ADD adult, society is ill equipped to manage this disorder. We deny or minimize the disorder's severity and impact. Still others view the disorder as a personal weakness. Because ADD is not as visually apparent as is the case with many physical disabilities, we tend to deny its existence.

Few employers know how to provide reasonable accommodations for ADD adults. Most ADD adults are completely unaware of their legal rights or entitlement to services and accommodations. As there are few legal precedents regarding ADD adults, most employers do not feel obligated to retain ADD employees. We need to strengthen legal avenues for the protection of ADD employees with legitimate concerns for accommodation.

Most ADD adults go undiagnosed. They have a direct impact on our society. I often wonder how many high school dropouts, as a result of unrecognized ADD, left school. How many of those same individuals have been repeatedly fired from employment or have turned to drugs and alcohol as a means of self-medicating. Left untreated, ADD symptoms do not improve.

In the schools, at some level, ADD is being addressed. Wanting a simple and easy solution, we quickly prescribe medication. It most cases, medication is a vital and necessary treatment; however, many educators still have unrealistic expectations as to what medication *will* or *will not* do. Without having a complete understanding of ADD, most teachers are unaware that even with medication, the disorder still exists. Although medication can significantly reduce symptoms, it does not cure the child of the disorder. Likewise, medication cannot cure learning disabilities. Educators should be open-minded with regard to finding new and creative ways to implement individual educational plans.

Educators should receive ongoing training in childhood disorders. Many children have more than one disorder, and often the symptoms of two or more of these disorders will overlap (co-morbidity). As many as two-thirds of children with ADD have one or more coexisting disorders. Most educators and many professionals receive little or no training on how to accurately diagnose ADD. As a result, some children are misdiagnosed.

Human service and social work agencies will inevitably employee ADD individuals. Most supervisors do not know how to manage an ADD employee. Many have transference issues, believing that only the clients and not the employees should be permitted to have this disorder. Supervisors and managers also lack the skills and knowledge necessary to effectively manage their ADD workers. Human Resources workers should be taught the fundamentals of job restructuring, understanding, and interpreting the Americans with Disabilities Act and learning how to harness the strengths and skills of its ADD workers. Work should be a place of advocacy not adversity.

Society will benefit from ongoing ADD research, including longitudinal studies. Availability and access to new data will aid in creating a greater public awareness of the disorder. Websites, seminars, conferences, newsletters, and symposiums all serve to further educate and disseminate this essential knowledge.

Fortunately, some advocacy and education is already occurring. Organizations like CHADD (Children and Adults With Attention-Deficit/Hyperactivity Disorder) are in the forefront of campaigning for greater public awareness and advocacy of children and adults with ADD. This not-for-profit organization has assisted in the funding for studies and research of ADD.

For those who have ADD, treatment is available. Medication has a proven and safe track record in treating adults with ADD. For those persons who struggle with living with ADD, this book has outlined numerous interventions and techniques that can assist in managing the disorder. As each person is unique, careful consideration should be given when deciding upon which interventions to employ. What may work for one individual may not work for another. There are no quick cookie-cutter solutions. Friends, family, and employers of people with ADD should listen to what the ADD person is saying and follow his lead regarding effective interventions. People with ADD can gain insight into their disorder. This can be a slow process. Patience and understanding is paramount for both the ADD individual and the people with whom he is living or working.

Parents should not become discouraged and worry about their ADD child's future. Some weaknesses can later become strengths. Be willing to place faith in the human potential. Considering the nature of his disability, my father's parents would never have imagined him in his chosen profession. My father, born in 1937, was born two months premature. His birth weight was slightly more than two pounds. In those days, the odds of surviving a premature birth were remote. He did survive, but had delayed speech. When he learned to speak, he stuttered. Throughout his childhood he would be plagued by this disorder. Since he struggled in articulating the English language, he decided to try his luck with another language. When speaking a foreign tongue, he did not stutter. Over time, he learned how to manage this disorder. Eventually he received his doctorate in foreign languages.

If you have ADD, don't become discouraged. Nobody's future is carved in stone. In many ways, your choices in managing ADD will positively influence your destiny. Don't become your biggest critic. Embrace your vicissitudes. Do not place limitations on yourself or allow others to place them upon you. Don't be ashamed of having ADD or a learning disability. Teach others what you know. Contribute to life and others will benefit from having you as part of their lives.

END

For more information on AD/HD contact:
National Resource Center on AD/HD
A program of CHADD
8181 Professional Place Suite 150
Landover MD, 20785
(800) 233-4050
<www.chadd.org>

EPILOGUE

I'm not exactly sure what constitutes a "successful" book, but I do know that if this small offering provides insight and symptom amelioration to even one person, I will be satisfied. If there is only one teacher who after reading this book is now more understanding of an ADD child, then that's a success. If there is a husband or wife who is now more informed about his or her ADD spouse, that's a success. If an ADD employee is able to sit down with his employer and in mutual dialogue discuss reasonable accommodations, then that too is a success.

In this book, I included only those stories and events that, in respect to my living with ADD, had the most direct impact and relevance. For example, I probably would have had to write an entirely separate book about my parenthood experiences. I love being a parent. When our oldest was born, the thought that I was now responsible for another human being's life seemed completely absurd. Nevertheless, my son is now seven years old, and my daughter is six. My wife continues her work as a day care preschool teacher. Every so often I can be found at a local club playing bass guitar with the band. As Neil Young once said, "Rock and roll will never die."

I continue working as a clinical manager in a residential setting, where I work with troubled adolescents who themselves have faced many difficulties. Their challenges help me keep things in perspective, as my hardships often are dwarfed in comparison. I am humbled yet inspired by the human spirit. Witnessing youth overcome adversity and rise above it is rewarding.

Being a supervisor brings many challenges. More recently, I am very fortunate to have had supervisors who are laid-back, flexible and amenable.

And whatever became of my best friend Steve? We still maintain contact with each other. Steve has had a successful career in the computer field. He is married with children. In respect to his history of tumultuous relationships, as the old saying goes, "The third time's a charm." And I think that at some level, I may have impacted *his* life. He married a social worker.

ACKNOWLEDGMENTS

Sometimes others touch our lives in ways that leave lasting impressions. In my life, this has certainly been the case. Certain individuals have unknowingly and inadvertently filled the pages of this book. They are the silent scribes and ghostwriters, and without their contributions, I could not have written this book.

I would like to thank the following individuals: Bryce Christensen for his constructive feedback, helping give the book clear parameters and greater clarity; Dr. Robert Eme for writing the book's foreword and making sure that the ADD data remained accurate; and Jean Campbell-Sooter for providing grammatical accuracy and vernacular clarity.

An expression of gratitude is also in order for Arizona State University's School of Social Work and the University of Illinois Graduate School of Social Work in Urbana/Champaign. In addition, I would like to thank Arizona State University's Disabled Student Services and Rockford College.

Writing can be challenging, and consequently I wish to thank my father, who painstakingly reviewed each chapter, and also my mother, who provided much of the early childhood history. A thank you to my wife and children, who graciously (well, maybe not my children) gave me time and space in which to write.

I owe a debt of gratitude to the Kjenners, the Gokeys, and the McConkies, who, during difficult times, remained my staunchest allies. Additionally, thank you to Nello Williams and John Copeland for introducing me to my respective musical instruments and teaching me how to play them.

Overseas, I am grateful for my Welsh maternal lineage, the Williams family, for their love of music and language.

Recognition is in order for my three sisters, who tolerated an ADD brother and had to accept the fact that I was the sibling who never had to share a bedroom, although with three sisters I saw very little of the bathroom.

And thanks to Doug Nelson, Steve Kjenner, Brian LeBaron, The MILL, and CHADD.

ABOUT THE AUTHOR

Ian Provo, MSW, LCSW, lives in Rockford, Illinois, with his wife, Heidi, and their two children. He is a clinician and clinical manager, whose diverse background and work experience includes, specialization in the treatment of child/adolescent behavioral disorders, mental illness, ADD, and marriage/family therapy.

www.ingramcontent.com/pod-product-compliance
Lightning Source LLC
Chambersburg PA
CBHW020431290526
45785CB00002B/802